BONE SCINTIGRAPHY

BOERHAAVE SERIES
FOR POSTGRADUATE
MEDICAL EDUCATION
Vol. 20

PROCEEDINGS OF BOERHAAVE COURSES
ORGANIZED BY
THE FACULTY OF MEDICINE, UNIVERSITY OF LEIDEN
THE NETHERLANDS

For complete series listing please refer to the last page in this book.

BONE SCINTIGRAPHY

edited by

ERNEST K.J. PAUWELS D.Sc.
University Hospital Leiden

HENRI E. SCHÜTTE M.D.
St. Elisabeth's of Groote Gasthuis Haarlem

WYBREN K. TACONIS M.D.
O.L. Vrouwe Gasthuis Amsterdam

Associate editor

PETER J. ELL M.D., M.Sc.
The Middlesex Hospital Medical School London

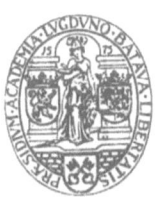

1981

LEIDEN UNIVERSITY PRESS

THE HAGUE/BOSTON/LONDON

Distributors:

for the United States and Canada

Kluwer Boston, Inc.
190 Old Derby Street
Hingham, MA 02043
USA

for all other countries

Kluwer Academic Publishers Group
Distribution Center
P.O. Box 322
3300 AH Dordrecht
The Netherlands

This volume is listed in the Library of Congress Cataloging in Publication Data

ISBN-13:978-94-009-8620-6   e-ISBN-13:978-94-009-8618-3
DOI: 10.1007/978-94-009-8618-3

CONTENTS

CONTRIBUTORS

Chris Alberts, M.D., Wilhelmina Gasthuis, University of Amsterdam, Eerste Helmersstraat 104, 1054 EG Amsterdam, The Netherlands.

Rodney G. Bessent, M.A., D.Phil., West of Scotland Health Boards, Department of Clinical Physics and Bio-engineering, Glasgow, Scotland, UK.

Peter J. Ell, M.D., M.Sc., Institute of Nuclear Medicine, The Middlesex Hospital Medical School, Mortimer Street, London W1N 8AA, UK.

Ignac Fogelman, M.B., Ch.B., M.R.C.P., University Departments of Medicine and Nuclear Medicine, Royal Infirmary, Glasgow G4 0SF, Scotland, UK.

Pieter de Graaf, M.D., Department of Nephrology, University Hospital Leiden, Rijnsburgerweg 10, 2333 AA Leiden, The Netherlands.

Paul B. Hoffer, M.D., Section of Nuclear Medicine, Yale University School of Medicine, 333 Cedar Street, New Haven, CT 06510, USA.

Peter H. Jarritt, B.Sc., Ph.D., Institute of Nuclear Medicine, The Middlesex Hospital Medical School, Mortimer Street, London W1N 8AA, UK.

Malcolm V. Merrick, M.D., Division of Nuclear Medicine, Western General Hospital, Edinburgh EH4 2XU, Scotland, U.K.

Barbara J. McNeil, M.D., Ph.D., Department of Radiology, Harvard Medical School, 25 Shattuck Street, Boston, MA 02115, USA.

Ernest K.J. Pauwels, D.Sc., Department of Diagnostic Radiology, Division of Nuclear Medicine, University Hospital Leiden, Rijnsburgerweg 10, 2333 AA Leiden, The Netherlands.

Joseph F. Polak, M.D., C.M., Department of Radiology, Harvard Medical School and the Joint Program in Nuclear Medicine, Peter Bent Brigham Hospital, Division of the Affiliated Hospitals Center, Inc., Boston, MA 02115, USA.

Robert Princenthal, M.D., The Milton S. Hershey Medical Center, The Pennsylvania State University, Hershey, PA 17033, USA.

Peter P. van Rijk, M.D., Institute of Nuclear Medicine. University Hospital Utrecht, Catharijnesingel 101, 3511 GV Utrecht, The Netherlands.

Rohit G. Radia, M.B., Ch.B., M.Med., M.Sc., Institute of Nuclear Medicine, The Middlesex Hospital Medical School, Mortimer Street, London W1N 8AA, UK.

Henri E. Schütte, M.D., Department of Radiology and Nuclear Medicine, St. Elisabeth's of Groote Gasthuis, Boerhaavelaan 22, 2035 RC Haarlem, The Netherlands.

Cees J.L.R. Vellenga, M.D., Department of Diagnostic Radiology, Prinses Irene Ziekenhuis, Boerhaavelaan 1, 7607 PW Almelo, The Netherlands.

Johan Vermey, M.D., Department of Radiotherapy, University Hospital Groningen, Oostersingel 59, 9713 EZ Groningen, The Netherlands.

PREFACE

This book is based on a series of lectures given by an international team as part of a course on Bone Scintigraphy organized by the Boerhaave Committe for Postgraduate Medical Education (Leiden, January 1980).

Bone scintigraphy and the use of radionuclide tracers in the investigation of skeletal pathology has developed into a subject of its own. Significant advances in instrumentation, radiopharmaceuticals and data analysis has considerably widened the scope of clinical application. Beyond the important area of sensitive detection of malignant involvement of the skeleton, major strides are being made in the investigation of benign bone disease and its metabolic aspects.

The structure of this Boerhaave Course reflects this change, with considerable emphasis being given to the discussion of recent methods for tracer uptake quantitation, the discussion of inflammatory osseous disease, benign pathology in general and the investigation of metabolic bone disease.

As a clinical tool, bone scintigraphy is present today in most if not all general and regional hospital institutions. It is a technique in demand by general interns, surgeons, radiologists, paediatricians, oncologists and radiotherapists. New areas of application are being evaluated and to some extent consolidated. These include the difficult orthopaedic issues of bone avascularity, prosthesis loosening, infection and non-apparent fractures. A range of new techniques are available and applied to the follow-up of osteomalacia, osteoporosis, osteodystrophy and other conditions where a more objective and even preferably a numerical approach is being explored. The inherent sensitivity of the radionuclide tracer method (despite its poor specificity) is a significant asset which is and will continue to be explored.

This book reviews a variety of topics, the aim being the dissemination of the clinical potential of bone scintigraphy.

The editors

PART I

TECHNOLOGY

1. RADIOPHARMACOLOGY OF BONE-SEEKING RADIOPHARMACEUTICALS AND SCINTIGRAPHIC IMAGING TECHNIQUES

ERNEST K.J. PAUWELS

Radiopharmacology
    properties of bone-seeking pharmaceuticals
    mechanism of bone uptake
Bone imaging equipment
    rectilinear scanning
    gamma camera

1. RADIOPHARMACOLOGY

1.1. *Introduction*

The widespread availability of artificially prepared radionuclides has prompted interdisciplinary efforts to develop radioactive compounds suitable for the evaluation of the skeletal system. The present status has been achieved by developments in the field of high resolution gamma cameras, in the knowledge of bone physiology, in the development of bone-seeking radiopharmaceuticals and in the knowledge of radiopharmacology of these radiotracers. Recently, a number of articles and oral presentations have contributed to the insight in the experimental and the clinical aspects of bone-seeking radiotracers. It is the purpose of this article to review these localization principles and other radiopharmacologic properties on the basis of results obtained in clinical and preclinical studies.

1.2. *Properties of bone-seeking radiopharmaceuticals*

The physical properties and nuclear characteristics of agents suitable for bone imaging are summarized in Table 1. For comparative reasons the obsolete radionuclide ^{85}Sr has been included. The agent was used often for clinical and experimental studies in the fifties and sixties, but is no longer applied in nuclear medicine bone studies.

Pauwels EKJ, Schütte HE, Taconis WK, eds, Bone scintigraphy, p 3–18.

Table 1. Characteristics of suitable bone-seeking agents for scintigraphic studies.

Radionuclide	Half-life	Photon energy (keV)	Mean beta energy (keV)	Administered. dose	Estimated radiation dose (rad/mCi) [a]	
					skeleton	red marrow
85Sr	64 days	514	0.014	0.1 mCi	31	11
87mSr	2.8 hr	388	0.082	1–5 mCi	0.15	0.5
18F	1.9 hr	511	0.28	2–5 mCi	0.18	0.4
135mBa	27.7 hr	268	0.25	5–10 mCi	1.3	0.3
153Sm [b]	47 hr	103	0.29	1 mCi	3.3	0.8
157Dy	8 hr	326	0.02	10 mCi	0.1	0.05
99mTc [c]	6 hr	140	0.014	10 mCi	0.04	0.03

[a] (1 rad/mCi = 0.27 Gy/GBq; 1 mCi = 37 MBq).
[b] Complexed with HEDTA.
[c] Average value for polyphosphate, pyrophosphate and diphosphonate.

It seems likely that the exchange for a hydroxyl or bicarbonate group in the crystalline hydroxyapatite is responsible for the localization of ^{18}F anion. The cationic radionuclides concentrate in bone due to the exchange with calcium of hydroxyapatite. The term "exchange" does not really indicate the "nature of the binding", as it has been proven that this binding may be reversible or irreversible. In the reversible process the radioactivity is extracted from blood into bone and returns to blood subsequently. Both for calcium and orthophosphate radioactive compounds, part of the activity may be bound to bone in a reversible way (1–3). The same compounds may also be bound in an irreversible way, as these physiological ions may be used in the synthesis of hydroxyapatite. This permanent fixation of radiotracers in newly formed bone is termed accretion (5). It seems logic to assume that the non-biological compounds listed in Table 1 bind to bone in a reversible manner, although it has been demonstrated that technetium-99m diphosphonate binds strongly to the hydroxyapatite crystal surface (6). Especially in the latter case, where the non-biologic entity technetium-diphosphonate is concentrated in bone, it seems more appropriate to use the term "absorption into bone surface" instead of "exchange with bone components". In case of absorption or reversible exchange reaction, the bone surface will most likely be the area where the tracer concentration takes place. This hypothesis is supported by autoradiographic work by Tilden et al. (4) and Guillemart et al. (8) (Figure 1).

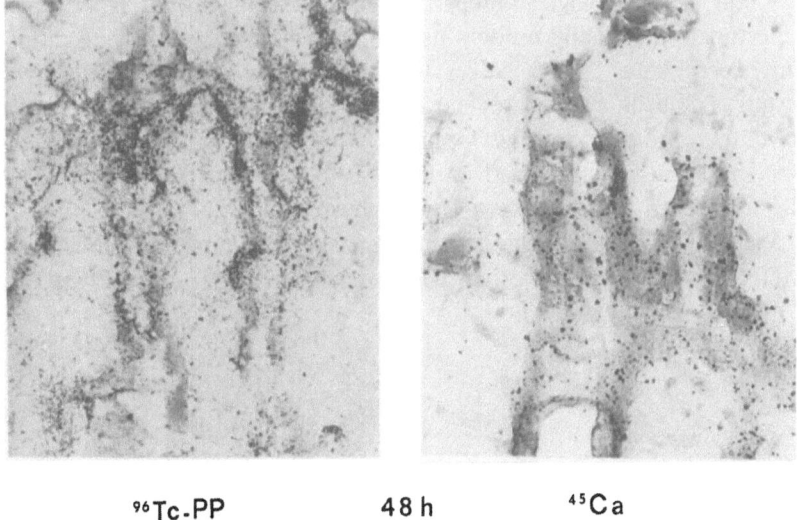

^{96}Tc-PP   48 h ^{45}Ca

Figure 1. Microautoradiographic studies in rabbit diaphysis showing calcium concentration in the calcium pool, whereas technetium-96 remains in linear deposits overlying osteoid structures. (reprinted from J Nucl Med 21:466-470, 1980).

6

Since the introduction of technetium-99m-labelled polyphosphate in 1971 by **Subramanian** (7) a considerable number of technetium-labelled phosphorus-containing compounds have been synthesized. Some of these compounds can be easily prepared with the aid of commercial kits, which are all based upon the reduction of ^{99m}Tc-pertechnetate by the stannous ion, present in the reaction vial as chloride, and the subsequent labelling of the phosphate moiety. The final preparation should have a slightly acid pH, as neutral or basic pH's tend to produce microcolloidal solutions as a probable result of hydroxide formation. The most relevant agents can chemically be classified in three different structures (Figure 2) including: 1) the P-O-P bond of the pyrophosphate and the larger chained polyphosphates, 2) the P-C-P bond of the diphosphonates with the strong non-hydrolyzable structure, and 3) the P-N-P bond of the imidodiphosphonates. Subramanian et al. (9) has pointed out that the structural formulas of pyrophosphate, methylene diphosphonate and imidodiphosphate are similar with respect to the interatomic P-P distance, which could be the basis of the bone-seeking properties. Comparison of commercially available radiopharmaceuticals for bone scintigraphy has revealed many data as to target/non-target ratios as a function of time after injection. The result of this work continuously shows the highest bone-to-background ratio for technetium-99m-labelled methylene diphosphonate (Tc-MDP). Recent experiments by Bevan et al. (10) have shown that the not commercially available compound technetium-99m-hydroxymethylene diphosphonate (Tc-HMDP) has still better biological properties for bone imaging. It is however unfortunate that many authors use different animal models and different experimental circumstances which hamper a clear comparison of results. Based on data by several authors and our own observations we have tried to compare the localization properties of various skeletal imaging agents (summarized in Table 2). Note again the superiority of the mentioned hydroxy methylene diphosphonate.

Visual comparison of the patient scans show the superiority of ^{99m}Tc-MDP images over the other commercially available agents. In our

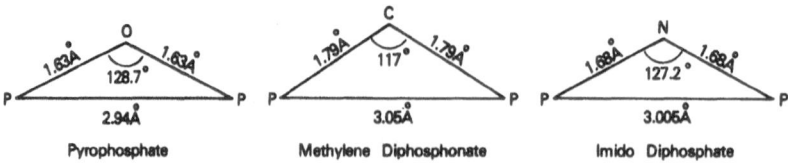

Figure 2. Structural formulas of three different phosphate-agents, showing similar interatomic P-P distances and bond angles (reprinted from J Nucl Med 16:1137-1143, 1975.

Table 2. Comparative results of approximate tissue concentration of various Technetium-99m-labelled bone-seeking agents at 3 hours after injection, in percent dose per gram tissue.

	Poly P	PPi	EHDP	MDP	HMDP
Femur	1.78	2.10	3.92	4.32	5.37
Blood	0.98	0.95	0.62	0.74	0.49
Muscle	0.19	0.18	0.10	0.11	0.07

Poly P = polyphosphate; PPi = pyrophosphate; EHDP = ethylane hydroxydiphosphonate; MDP = methylenediphosphonate; HMDP = hydroxymethylene diphosphonate.

experience, however, we often find it difficult to make technically adequate scintiphoto's with MDP, especially in children, due to the relatively high bone uptake, which easily causes oversaturation of the image. The agent is clearly superior in obese patients, but for daily routine we prefer ^{99m}Tc-EHDP. Moreover, it has been shown by Fogelman (37, 38) that the tumour/bone ratio for Tc-EHDP is slightly higher than for Tc-MDP and Tc-PPi. The biologic characteristics of ^{18}F make it the ideal agent for bone imaging due to its fast blood clearance, high skeletal uptake and low radiation dose. Although some commercial sources have made Fluorine-18 available in the past, the cyclotron-produced agent has never gained popularity over the cheap ^{99m}Technetium-phosphate compounds, which are readily available in every nuclear medicine institution. The almost ideal characteristics of the ^{99m}Tc-phosphate complexes can be summarized as follows:

1. low radiation dose to bone and bone marrow.
2. readily available in kit form.
3. production on instant basis with generator-produced ^{99m}Tc.
4. low cost per patient examination.
5. easy quality control.
6. high bone uptake and low soft tissue and blood activity.
7. high resolution image with present gamma cameras.

As is shown in Figure 3 the blood concentration of the radioactivity does not change much further after $2-2\frac{1}{2}$ hours. To allow adequate soft tissue clearance a waiting time of 3 hours is usually required. After this period adequate scintiphotos can be obtained with an initial dose of 10 mCi (370 MBq) for adult patients. By curve analysis it is demonstrated that blood clearance of ^{99m}Tc-phosphorous complexes is essentially tri-exponential. The first, most rapid, component (75% of the

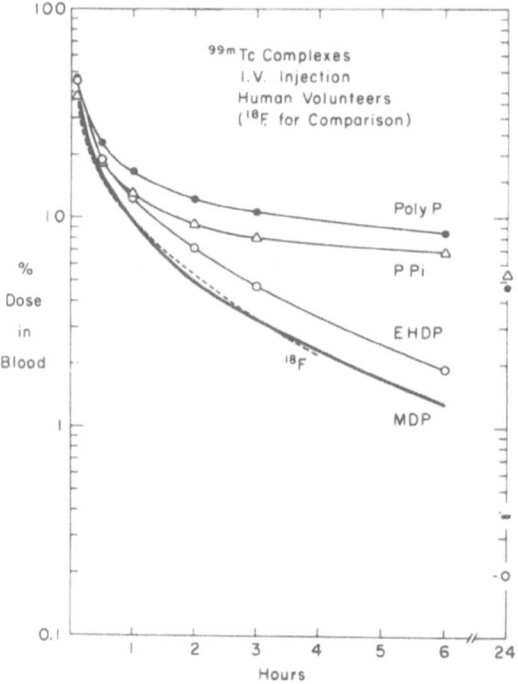

Figure 3. Bloodclearance of ^{99m}Tc-labelled phosphate agents and ^{18}F in humans (reprinted from J Nucl Med 16:744-755, 1975).

injected dose) has a half-life of 4–6 minutes and presumably represents the distribution of the radiotracer between blood and extracellular fluid. The second component (20% of the injected dose) most likely represents the bone uptake and has a half-life of around 30 minutes. The third component (5% of the injected dose) is believed to reflect the renal clearance of the fraction of radioactivity remaining in the blood after the first two disappearance processes are completed. The half-life time of the last component is dependant of the radiopharmaceutical and basically determines the visual appearance of the bone scintigraphic image. Although considerable differences between the various agents are appreciated, it is the author's experience that bone scans made with the mentioned phosphorous containing agents, all show bone lesions in a qualitatively similar manner, which is reassuring for the clinician, who is directly, or indirectly involved in bone scintigraphy.

A new and perhaps promising development in the application of bone-seeking radiopharmaceuticals is described by Cox et al. (11) who found a higher detection rate for bone metastases with the use of ^{99m}Tc-polyphosphate than with other ^{99m}Tc-phosphate compounds. This phenomenon may be associated with the presence of a relatively high amount of colloid in the polyphosphate preparation, which leads to augmented uptake in areas of increased histiocyte activity in the metastatic bone lesion. Especially in those cases where bone mineral is less affected, this mechanism might explain the enhanced uptake in lesions not observed with, for instance, ^{99m}Tc-MDP.

Occasionally ^{67}Ga-citrate is used for bone scintigraphy. The role of Ga-scanning for bone tumours is almost nil, although some applications are mentioned (12). The radiopharmaceutical has, on the other hand, an important place in the detection of infectious bone disease, which is reviewed in this book in the chapter on inflammatory bone disease.

The localization mechanism of gallium in the inflammatory lesion has been the subject of many studies. There is some evidence that bacteria themselves, as is the case in Staphylococcus Aureus, may accumulate the radioisotope (13). Also, experiments have been performed which establish the location of ^{67}Ga in lysosomes (14), the uptake being dependant on the lysosomal enzyme activity (15, 17). In addition, the resemblance of gallium to iron has made it plausible that ^{67}Ga, taken up by leucocytes, binds to lactoferrin, which is present in increased concentrations in leucocyte surrounding exudates (16). Although the exact mechanism by which the localization of ^{67}Ga takes place is unclear, the radiopharmaceutical has proven to be very helpful in the diagnosis of inflammatory bone disease, due to the high concentration of polymorphonuclear leucocytes in the affected area.

1.3. *Mechanism of bone uptake of ^{99m}technetium-phosphorous complexes*

A high concentration of these agents is found in the vicinity of bone lesions. This phenomenon is currently ascribed to processes associated with increased blood flow, increased surface area, reactive bone formation, increased capillary permeability and metabolic action.

However, in an excellent review paper by Charkes (18) it is pointed out that an increased blood flow through normally patent vessels does not considerably add to an increased tracer uptake at the pathologic area. Within the concept of " diffusion-limited flow " it is explained that the tracer may rapidly enter the extracellular space which surrounds the osteoid surface, but its transfer to bone is a slow process more or less controlled by diffusion laws. Under pathologic conditions such as fracture, infection or tumour involvement, loss of neurogenic control may cause an hyperaemic effect by the opening of normally closed arterioles ("recruitment"). This augmented blood flow may cause the area of increased activity in and around the bone lesion. Experimental evidence for this model is also given by Citrin et al. in 1975(19), who have shown that bone uptake in normal bone is a biexponential process with a fast component of about 12 minutes half-life time and a slow component with a half-life of about 53 minutes. It is interesting to speculate whether the first component may be the transfer into the mentioned extracellular fluid and the second component the diffusion controlled uptake in bone. It was further noted that a continuing increase of tracer uptake takes place in the tumour area, which can be explained by the local hyperaemia, facilitating and increasing tracer contact with osteoid surfaces. In addition to this blood flow phenomenon, increased tracer concentration is almost invariably caused by osseous repair. With respect to this uptake mechanism it is believed that the accumulation of [99m]technetium-phosphorous complexes (a) takes place onto the hydroxy-apatite crystal, (b) is associated with immature collagen or (c) finds its origin in enzymatic inhibition.

a. *Uptake in hydroxyapatite.* Microautoradiographic studies by Van Langevelde et al. (20) and Guillemart et al. (8) have shown that ^{99m}Tc-phosphorous complexes may well localize onto bone-crystal nuclei (Figure 1). According to Francis et al. (6) and Jones et al. (21) radiotracer uptake occurs primarily in inorganic bone, preferably at sites of mineralization where small nuclei of calcium phosphate are being formed. It is postulated (20) that the bond between EHDP and bone is stronger than that between technetium and its ligands. Once the radiopharmaceutical has arrived at the bone surface this difference in binding permits technetium to bind directly to bone. Thus the diphosphonate would only act as a carrier for the radioisotope on its way to the bone surface. This hypothesis of independant binding of free reduced technetium species is supported by experiments by Tofe and Francis (22) who suggested that EHDP and free reduced technetium compete for the binding sites at the bone surface.

b. *Uptake in immature collagen.* In a study by Tilden et al. (4) it was demonstrated that silver granules representing radioactivity after injection with ^{99m}Tc-polyphosphate were localized in bone areas which appeared more immature than surrounding bone. In an elegant study with ^{32}P-pyrophosphate, ^{14}C-diphosphonate and ^{99m}Tc-labelled polyphosphate, pyrophosphate and EHDP in rats with induced rickets (25), it could be shown that the technetium labelled compounds concentrated in the inorganic and organic bone components, whereas the ^{32}P and ^{14}C activity was mainly found in the inorganic phase. In view of these results it seems likely that the technetium-phosphorous complex is preferentially bond by immature collagen. Wiegmann et al. (23) have correlated bone uptake of Tc-pyrophosphate and hydroxyproline in blood and urine of uremic patients. Also on the basis of their observations in hyperparathyroidism (24) it is suggested that elevated uptake of the Tc-phosphate moiety reflects an excess of immature collagen characteristic of osteomalacia. In further studies with uremic patients in a state of renal osteodystrophy, de Graaf et al. (26) have pointed out that defective mineralization results in increased quantities of immature collagen and the presence of amorphous calcium-phosphate. It is therefore conceivable that the increased bone uptake in these metabolic bone diseases may well be attributed to both binding by immature collagen and growing calcium-phosphate nuclei.

c. *Uptake by enzymatic inhibition.* Contrary to the hypothesis that Tc-99m labelled phosphorous complexes are localized by binding to hydroxyapatite crystals or immature collagen, there has been some evidence that the radiotracer accumulates by combining with enzymes. Both alkaline and acid phosphatase is inactivated by adequate amounts of ^{99m}Tc-EHDP (27). By adding calcium or magnesium ions to the inactivated enzyme-EHDP complex, the enzyme could be reactivated completely, presumably by recomplexing of EHDP by the cations and thereby releasing free phosphatase. The enzyme-receptor binding of ^{99m}Tc-diphosphonate might well explain the localization of technetium phosphorous compounds in breast tumours that show no microscopic calcification but high concentration of acid phosphatase (27). In addition it could be an explanation for the accumulation of ^{99m}Tc-pyrophosphate in the acute myocardial infarct, the intensity of uptake in the infarcted area being almost proportional to the patients serum enzyme response (28). Due to the ruptured necrotic cell wall Tc-EHDP might be bound by enhanced extracellular enzyme concentration or by faciliated binding to intracellular enzymes.

High concentration of alkaline and acid phosphatase are found in areas of pathologic bone. This increased enzyme concentration may account for the increased technetium radioactivity in abnormal bone. The controversial validity of this theory is illustrated by the fact that in parathyroid disease a good correlation was found between alkaline phosphatase and overall bone uptake by de Graaf et al. (26), whereas such a relation could not be found by Wiegmann et al. (24) and Krishnamurthy et al. (29). Further difficulties arose with the observations by Rohlin et al. (30), who found no evidence that tissue uptake of ^{99m}Tc-labelled pyrophosphate depends on the activity of alkaline phosphatase in intestinal mucosa.

In summary we believe that at present few conclusions about the uptake mechanism can be drawn. Clear proof for enzyme contribution in the trapping of the technetium-phosphate moiety is lacking. The substantial evidence of binding to either hydroxyapatite or immature collagen makes one suppose that both processes may actually take place. The formation of hydroxyapatite and collagen are well related and may certainly both contribute to the localization process of these radiopharmaceuticals.

2. BONE IMAGING EQUIPMENT

Most of the commercially available equipment is optimized to the imaging of ^{99m}Tc and its radiopharmaceuticals. Only a few rectilinear scanners are equipped with crystals and extra shielding for the efficient and optimal detection of radiotracers with high photon energies (such as strontium-85 and fluorine-18). Routine imaging with technetium-99m labelled phosphates is done with Anger type gamma cameras and collimators, that are sensitive and yield high resolution bone images.

For the investigation of benign bone disease (such as inflammation or trauma), it is usually sufficient to image the skeletal segment involved. For such purposes the gamma camera or the rectilinear scanner are suitable apparatus. For other purposes, it can be very useful to record the whole skeleton. This is especially true for the tracing and evaluation of bone metastases and other skeletal abnormalities which may be present in multiple skeletal segments. As many excellent reviews about nuclear medicine instrumentation have been published in the past (31–36) the reader is referred to these for more extensive and detailed information. The purpose of the underlying text is to give a brief outline of the apparatus used for bone imaging.

2.1. *Rectilinear scanning*

Dual head scanners with one scintillation crystal above the patient and another crystal under the patient may be designed as organ scanners or whole body scanners. In the latter case their field range covers an area of at least 60×200 cm. For practical reasons the image of a whole body scanner is minified to 1/4 or 1/5 of the actual skeletal size.

Dual head scanners allow for the simultaneous registration of the ventral and dorsal view of the skeleton, and also for the recording of studies with radionuclides emitting photons of 300 keV or even higher energy, such as ^{67}Ga and ^{131}I. With the use of focussing collimators it is important to adjust the position of both detectors according to the focus characteristics and body contours of the patient. A recent development consists of an array of ten scintillation crystals—each with its own focussed collimator and electronics—in one detector head above the patient and in a second detector head underneath (Figure 4).

While the detector heads (60 cm wide) move over the patient in a cranio-caudal direction, the crystal array makes an oscillating motion in the lateral direction. For this type of imaging special collimators were developed providing a long and narrow cigar-shaped focus. This type of linear scanner is obviously much faster than the conventional rectilinear scanner. In our experience a two sided whole body image can be obtained in 30 minutes with a clinically sufficient resolution. However, in our hands it proved to be useful to repeat certain equivocal areas with the gamma camera in order to get the highest resolution possible. As the practical use of this machine is limited to the imaging of the whole body, it may only have a place in those institutions where a high patient load of bone examination exists. In such departments the semi-automatic character of the apparatus allows up to 15 bone scans a day with minimal personnel effort.

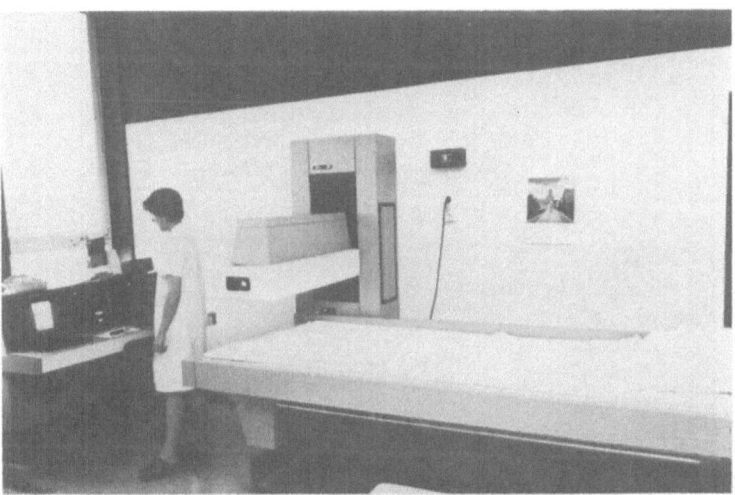

Figure 4. Dual Head detector scanner (Cleon) with arrays of 10 detectors above and 10 detectors under the patient. The detector heads move over the patient.

14

2.2. *Gamma camera imaging*

Multiple views can be taken with a gamma camera and this provides a survey of the whole skeleton, in which the resolution of the gamma camera is fully utilized. With the present large-field gamma camera with a 35-40 cm field size, a whole body composite image can be obtained with 8-10 static scintigrams. According to the dose administered and the technician's skill the study takes 45-60 minutes.

A widely used alternative to static imaging is the whole body imaging in which either the detector head moves over the table with the patient or the table moves under the detector head (Figure 5). All these systems allow for the camera to be positioned under the table with the collimator facing upwards. The dual view of the skeleton may be obtained in one to three automatically performed longitudinal scans in order to cover the width of the patient. A complete study takes 30–50 minutes and offers a good alternative for the linear scanner mentioned above.

The advantages of the gamma camera and the linear scanner have been combined in a new development, known as the multiplane tomographic scanner (Figure 6). A dual-head gamma camera detector with focussed collimators moves over and beneath the patient. The design allows the tomographic imaging at planes at six different distances from one collimator. Thus, a complete study viewing the ventral and dorsal

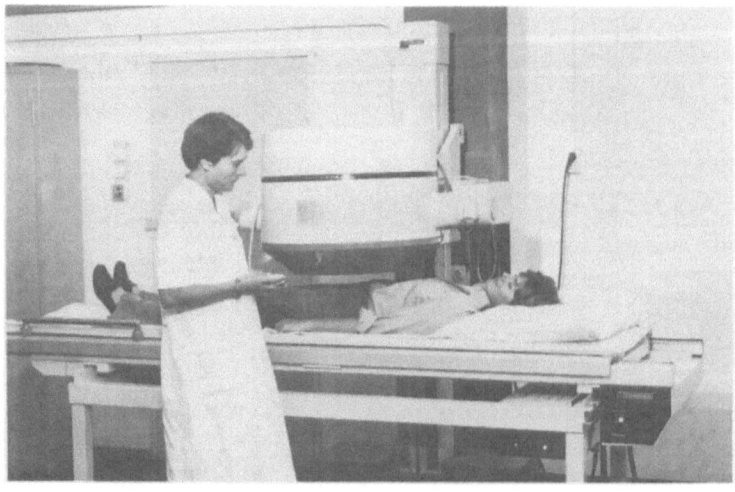

Figure 5 a. Whole body bed device (Toshiba) with patient moving under gamma camera in two or three automatically performed longitudinal movements.

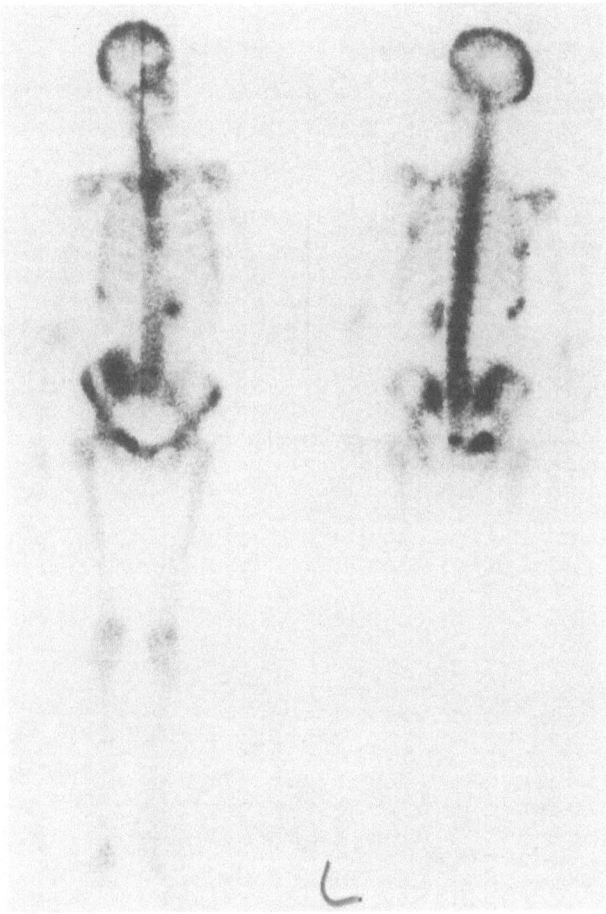

Figure 5b. Whole body bone scan (left: frontal view, right: dorsal view), made with gamma camera and moving bed. Note the "zipper" phenomenon resulting from the electronic combination of two separate longitudinal movements.

side of the patient contains twelve images. The dots on the various scintigrams are arranged in a way that only the structures at a certain depth are in focus, while structures at other levels appear out of focus. This scanner provides high spatial resolution at all tomographic levels and therefore offers a considerable advantage over the other scanning systems mentioned above.

Finally, it need be said that certain studies require quantitative assessment of the amount of radioactivity present in the bone. Such examinations use dedicated computers and are most often performed in association with gamma cameras.

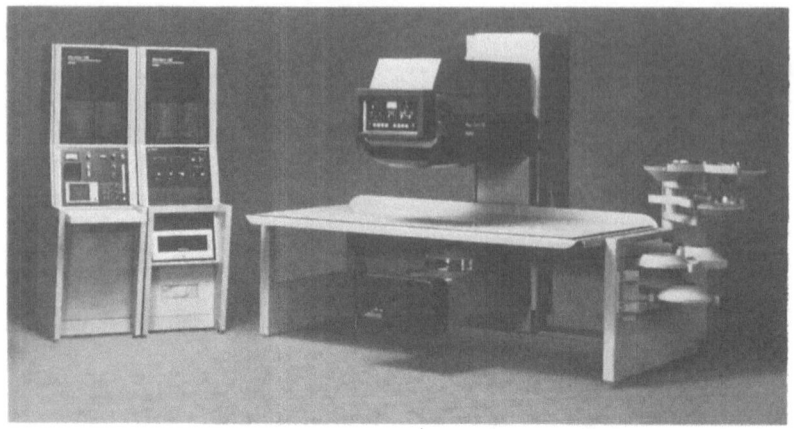

Figure 6a. Multiplane tomographic scanner with dual head and image control desk (courtesy Searle Radiographics).

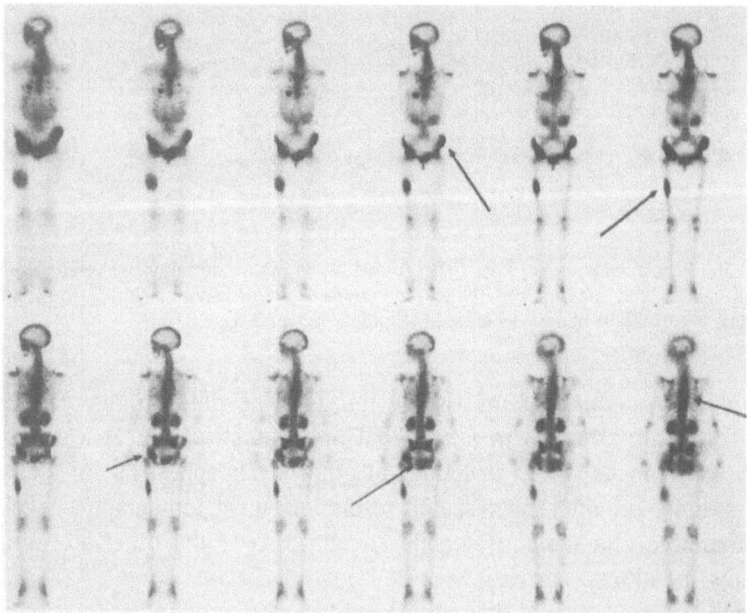

Figure 6b. Simultaneous tomograms of the skeleton obtained with the multiplane tomographic scanner, showing bone lesions at various depths in the body (courtesy J.A. Burdine, Houston, Tx, USA).

REFERENCES

1. Arnold JS, Jee WSS: Ion exchange and recrystallization in fixation of ^{45}Ca in the rabbit's skeleton. Proc Soc Exp Biol Med 85:658-663, 1954.
2. Neuman WF, Neuman MW: The nature of the mineral phase of bone. Chem Rev 53:1-45, 1953.
3. Rowland RE: Exchangeable bone calcium. Clin Orthop Rel Res 49:233-248, 1966.
4. Tilden RL, Jackson J, Enneking WF, DeLand FH, McVey JT: ^{99m}Tc-polyphosphate: histological localization in human femurs by autoradiography. J Nucl Med 14:576-578, 1973.
5. Carolsson A: Metabolism of radiocalcium in relation to calcium intake in young rats. Acta Pharmacol Toxicol 7:3-74, (suppl 1) 1951.
6. Francis MD, Tofe AJ, Benedict JJ, Bevan JA: Imaging the skeletal system. In: Proceedings 2nd International Symposium on Radiopharmaceuticals, Seattle, Society of Nuclear Medicine (ed), New York, 1979, p 603-614.
7. Subramanian G, McAfee JG, O'Mara Re, Rosenstreich M, Mehter A: ^{99m}Tc-polyphosphate PP46: A new radiopharmaceutical for skeletal imaging. J Nucl Med 12:399-400, 1971.
8. Guillemart A, Besnard J-C, Le Pape A, Galy G, Fetissoff F: Skeletal uptake of pyrophosphate labeled with technetium-95m and technetium-96, as evaluated by autoradiography. J Nucl Med 19:895-899, 1978.
9. Subramanian G, McAfee JG, Blair RJ, Rosenstreich M, Coco M, Duxbury CE: Technetium-99m-labeled stannous imidodiphosphate, a new radiodiagnostic agent for bone scanning: comparison with other ^{99m}Tc complexes. J Nucl Med 16:1137-1143, 1975.
10. Bevan JA, Tofe AJ, Francis MD, Barnet BL, Benedict JJ: Tc-99m-hydroxymethylene diphosphonate (HMDP): A new skeletal imaging agent. In: Proceedings 2nd International Symposium on Radiopharmaceuticals, Seattle, Society of Nuclear Medicine (ed), New York, p 645-654.
11. Cox PH, Belfer AJ, Van Dongen DJ, Perlberger R, Treurniet RE: The clinical reliability of ^{99m}Tc-polyphosphate skeletal scintigraphy in the early detection of bone metastases. Eur J Nucl Med 2:43-46, 1977.
12. Ito Y, Nagai K, Otsuka N, Yamashita K, Yokobayashi T, Muanaka A, Terashima H: Experimental and clinical studies on differential diagnosis of bone diseases with nucleo medical procedures. Eur J Nucl Med 5:357-368, 1980.
13. Menon S, Wagner HN, Tsan MF: Studies on gallium accumulation in inflammatory lesions: II. Uptake by staphylococcus aureus: concise communication. J Nucl Med 19:44-47, 1978.
14. Swartzendruber DC, Nelson B, Hayes RL: Gallium-67 localization in lysosome-like granules of leukaemic and nonleukaemic murine tissues. J Natl Cancer Inst 46:941-952, 1971.
15. Hammersley PAG, Taylor DM: The role of lysosomal enzyme activity in the localization of ^{67}gallium citrate. Eur J Nucl Med 4: 261-270, 1979.
16. Wright DG, Pizzo PA, Jones AE, Greenwald D, Deisserath AB: Studies of ^{67}Ga uptake at sites of neutrophil exudation. Clin Res 27:360A, 1979.
17. Hammersley PAG, Taylor DM: The mechanism of the localization of ^{67}gallium citrate in experimental abscesses. Eur J Nucl Med 4:271-275, 1979.
18. Charkes ND: Skeletal blood flow: implication for bone scan interpretation. J Nucl Med 21:91-98, 1980.
19. Citrin DL, Bessent RG, McGinley E, Gordon D: Dynamic studies with ^{99m}Tc-HEDP in normal subjects and in patients with bone tumors. J Nucl Med 16:886-890, 1975.
20. Van Langevelde A, Driessen OMJ, Pauwels EKJ, Thesing CW: Aspects of ^{99m}technetium binding from an ethane-1-hydroxy-1,1-diphosphonate-^{99m}Tc complex to bone. Eur J Nucl Med 2:47-51, 1977.

18

21. Jones AG, Francis MD, Davis MA: Bonescanning: radionuclide reaction mechanisms. Semin Nucl Med 6:no. 1, 3-18, 1976.
22. Tofe AJ, Francis MD: Optimization of the ratio of stannous tin: ethane-1-hydroxy-1, 1-diphosphonate for bone scanning with ^{99m}Tc-pertechnetate. J Nucl Med 15:69-74, 1974.
23. Wiegmann T, Kirsh J, Rosenthall L, Kaye M: Relationship between bone uptake of ^{99m}Tc-pyrophosphate and hydroxyproline in blood and urine. J Nucl Med 17:711-714, 1976.
24. Wiegmann T, Rosenthall L, Kaye M: Technetium-99m pyrophosphate bone scans in hyperparathyroidism. J Nucl Med 18:231-235, 1977.
25. Kaye M, Silverton S, Rosenthall L: Technetium-99m-pyrophosphate: studies in vivo and in vitro. J Nucl Med 16:40-45, 1975.
26. De Graaf P, Te Velde J, Pauwels EKJ, Schicht IM, Kleiverda K, De Graeff J: Increased bone radiotracer uptake in renal osteodystrophy. Eur J. Nucl Med 1980 (in press).
27. Zimmer AM, Isitman AT, Holmes RA: Enzymatic inhibition of diphosphonate: A proposed mechanism of tissue uptake. J Nucl Med 16:352-356, 1975.
28. Coleman RE, Klein MS, Roberts R, Sobel BE: Improved detection of myocardial infarction with technetium-99m stannous pyrophosphate and serum MB creatine phosphokinase. Am J Cardiol 37:732-735, 1976.
29. Krishnamurthy GT, Brickman AS, Blahd WH: Technetium-99m-Sn-pyrophosphate pharmaco-kinetics and bone image changes in parathyroid disease. J Nucl Med 18:236-242, 1977.
30. Rohlin M, Larsson A, Hammarström L: In vitro interaction between ^{99m}Tc-labelled pyrophosphate, ^{32}P-labelled pyrophosphate and rat tissues. Eur J Nucl Med 3:249-255, 1978.
31. Harbert JC, Neto AD: Rectilinear scanners. In: Textbook of nuclear medicine: basic science, Rocha AFG, Harbert JC (eds), Philadelphia, Lea and Febiger, 1978, p 249-263.
32. Erickson JJ, Brill AB: Scintillation cameras. In: Textbook of nuclear medicine: basic Science, Rocha AFG, Harbert JC (eds), Philadelphia, Lea and Febiger, 1978, P 264-284.
33. Parker Rp, Smith PHS, Taylor DM: Basic science of nuclear medicine; Part III, measurement and instrumentation, p 149-236, Edinburgh, Churchill Livingstone, 1978.
34. Early PJ, Razzak MA, Sodee DB: Textbook of Nuclear Medicine Technology, St. Louis, The C.V. Mosby Co, 1975.
35. Hine GJ, Erickson JJ: Advances in scintigraphic instruments. In: Instrumentation in nuclear medicine, Hine GJ, Sorenson JA (eds), New York and London, Academic Press, 1974, p 1-59.
36. Freeman LM, Blaufox MD: Recent advances in nuclear imaging instrumentation. Semin Nucl Med 7:no. 4, 263-281, 1977.
37. Fogelman I, Citrin DL, McKillop JH, Turner JG, Bessent RG, Greig WR: A clinical comparison of Tc-99m HEDP and Tc-99m MDP in the detection of bone metastases: concise communication. J Nucl Med 20:98-101, 1979.
38. Fogelman I, McKillop JH, Citrin DL: A clinical comparison of ^{99m}Tc-hydroxyethylidene-diphosphonate (H.E.D.P.) and ^{99m}Tc-pyrophosphate in the detection of bone metastases. Clin Nucl Med 2:364-367, 1977.

2. PITFALLS IN BONE SCINTIGRAPHY

PETER P. VAN RIJK

Normal scintigram
Pseudo normal scintigram
Decreased uptake ("cold spot", "photon deficient area")
Increased uptake ("hot spot")

1 INTRODUCTION

The breakthroughs by Subramanian and others (1–3) which led to the currently used ^{99m}Tc-labeled bone imaging agents can be regarded as a major success of nuclear medicine. The use of these compounds results in many advantages over the earlier imaging agents—the most important being lower patient radiation dose, immediate availability, lower cost, better bone-to-soft tissue visualization and physical characteristics more suitable for imaging with current-generation gamma cameras. The scintigrams are accepted as an extremely sensitive indicator of osseous pathology, although they have poor specificity. However, if the overall pattern of the normal scintigram is understood, it is possible to identify and interpret the disease process involved, particularly where the entire skeleton has been included in the study. Unexpected abnormalities can be introduced into the scintigram which results in false negative and false positive outcomes. Several of these pitfalls will be described, but first the appearance of the normal scintigram will be characterized.

2. NORMAL SCINTIGRAM

In the posterior view the larger part of the radioactivity is seen over the entire spine and sacroiliac joints. Iliac wings, ischial tuberosities and posterior skull are also best seen on this projection. Uptake in the cervical spine should never equal or exceed that of the dorsal and lumbar spine. The inferior tips of the scapulae frequently show up clearly, sometimes asymmetrically, and should not be confused with

Pauwels EKJ, Schütte HE, Taconis WK, eds, Bone scintigraphy, p 19–34.
Copyright © 1981 Martinus Nijhoff Publishers bv, The Hague/Boston/London. All rights reserved.

osseous disease. Anteriorly, most of the radioactivity is usually seen in the sternum and anterior iliac spine with clavicles, anterior skull, facial bones and pubic rami showing up clearly. Intermediate structures such as shoulders and hips are usually equally well visualized on both views. The skull uptake is extremely variable, ranging from an intensity as great as that seen in the spine to less than that seen in long bones. The facial bones demonstrate a high increase of radioactivity, probably due to the well vascularized structures and excretion of pertechnetate into the nasopharyngeal area.

The pubic symphysis is mostly obscured by radioactive urine in the bladder. In children and adolescents the normal pattern is different; there is an intense uptake of the radiopharmaceutical in regions of growth, causing sharp, clear delineation of epiphyseal plates. (Figure 1)

3. PSEUDO-NORMAL SCINTIGRAMS

In a large series of bone scintigrams an extremely low false negative rate was reported (less than 10%)(4). Several factors, however, have been reported to be associated with false negative scintigrams, of which a number can easily be recognized if the observer considers the clinical data available:

Metabolic bone disorders. Abnormal bone collagen metabolism is a feature of osteomalacia, Paget's disease, hyperparathyroidism (Figure 2) and renal osteodystrophy. In most cases, except for Paget's disease which shows localized defects, a diffuse elevated uptake of the tracer is registered (5–7), which can easily be misinterpreted as normal. One striking aspect of most of these scintigrams, viz. the absent kidney sign (see Figure 3), helps to avoid this pitfall.

Diffuse symmetric metastatic disease. The bone scintigrams of patients with a diffuse metastatic disease will create serious problems for the investigator, particularly if he is unaware of the presence of this disease. The scintigram will appear as an perfectly normal scan or even as a "super" scintigram in which all the bone structures are clearly visible. However upon more careful examination an "unbalanced" deposition of the radiopharmaceutical over the skeleton can be seen (Figure 4). In cases of a high uptake this can result in an absent kidney sign.

Drug therapy. Medical treatment for coexisting diseases, especially large doses of corticosteroids or antibiotics, may produce confusing images. Large doses of steroids will cause a decalcification of the skeleton and the scintigrams are similar as those obtained from patients with osteoporosis. Sometimes fractures occur while the scintigram

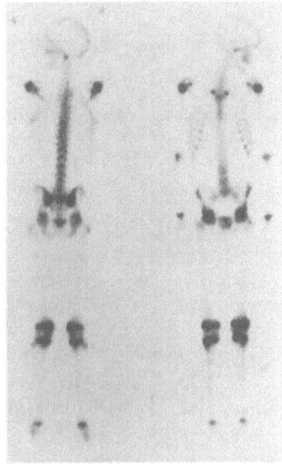

Figure 1. Normal scintigram of a fourteen-year-old male. A marked increase of radioactivity over the areas of the epiphyseal plates can be noted.

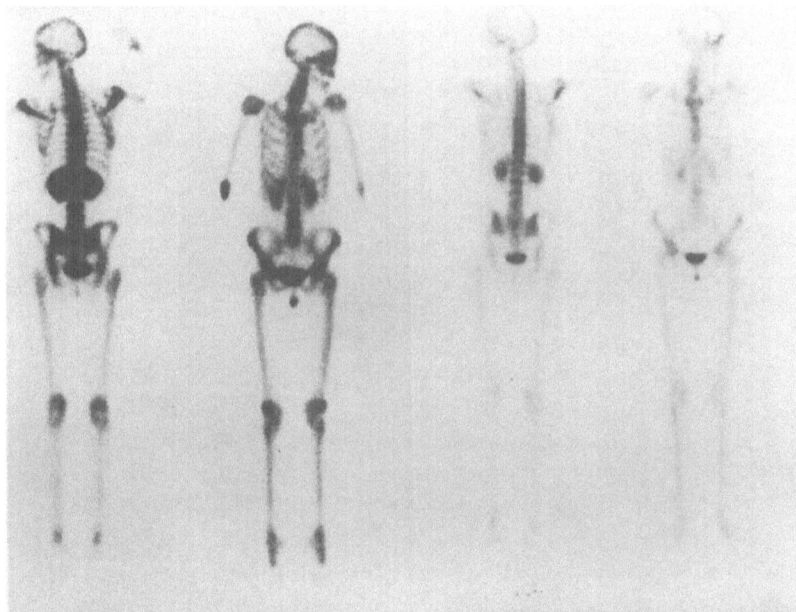

Figure 2. Bone scintigrams of a patient with hyperparathyroidism before and after treatment. Before treatment an extensive increase of radioactivity over the whole skeleton can be seen while after treatment the scintigrams return to normal.

The bone scintigrams before and after treatment were made under the same conditions, e.g.: amount of radioactivity administered and same camera setting.

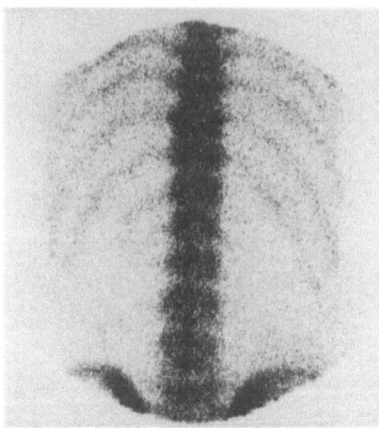

Figure 3. Typical example of a case with a metabolic bone disorder. This scintigram is pseudo-normal because the "absent kidney sign" points at an abnormality.

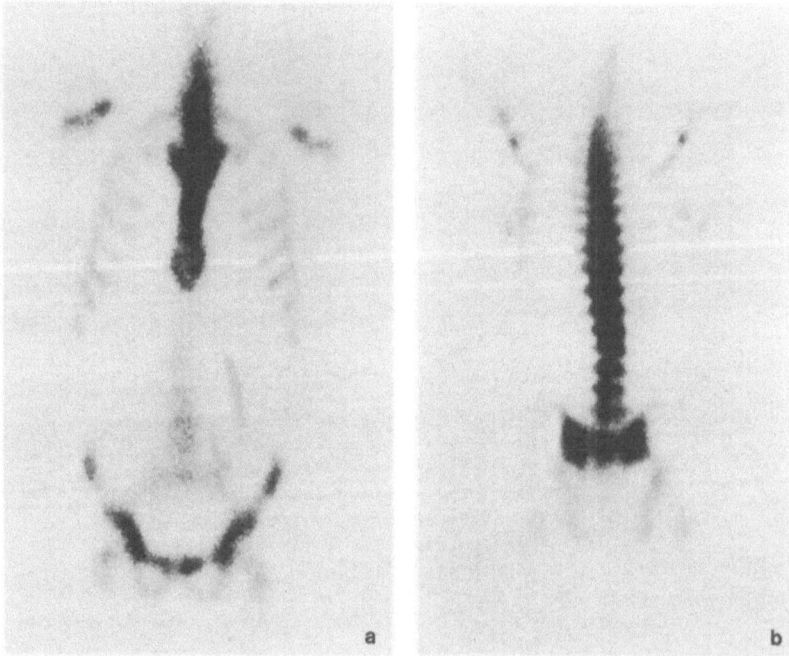

Figure 4. Anterior and posterior view of a bone scintigram of a patient with a symmetric diffuse metastatic disease of unknown origin.

No hot spots can be seen, however "unbalanced" deposition of the radioactivity with high uptake over the spine, sternum and iliac wings exists.

remains negative due to the extensive bone resorption. In inflammatory osseous diseases, especially acute osteomyelitis, it is well known that a relatively large percentage of the bone scans appears normal. In infants the incidence of negative scans can be even higher. Quite often medical therapy is started shortly after onset of pain and this can obscure the images.

4. DECREASED UPTAKE AREAS

Scintigrams with areas of decreased uptake are seldom seen. In most instances they are due to one of the following causes and are easily recognized as such:

Artefacts. The most common cause of abnormal scintigrams are pieces of metal in the pocket of patients e.g. coins, purses, keys, etc. In some scintigrams of female patients one can detect a decreased activity over the neck region, due to an ornament (see Figure 5). All these findings are easily detectable, but a breastprothesis or a "lunch syndrome" (9) can pass unnoticed.

Radiotherapy. High radiation dose levels delivered to bone may initially produce variable uptake, but eventually consistently produce marked decrease in osteoblastic activity and radionuclide incorporation into bone for long periods of time (10, 11) (see Figure 6).

Osteolytic defects. Fast growing metastases, in which the osteoclastic activity dominate, show up as cold areas in the scintigram.

5. INCREASED UPTAKE AREAS

Routinely, the observer is searching for areas of increased activity, knowing a wide range of bone disorders show an elevated uptake. Occasionally the scintigrams are misinterpreted, which results in false positive conclusions. Again, several easily recognizable factors are associated with these pitfalls and can be separated from the real skeletal diseases.

Artefacts. The most common artefact seen in bone scintigraphy is a hot spot at the site of injection. This usually does not result in errors in interpretation. A more serious cause of hot spots is contamination with urine or a contaminated handkerchief (Figure 7). In these cases one must not hesitate to repeat the study after having cleaned the involved area.

24

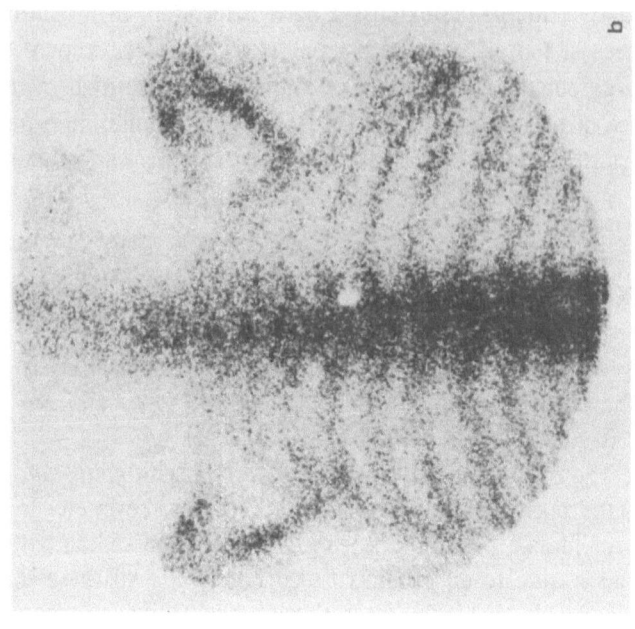

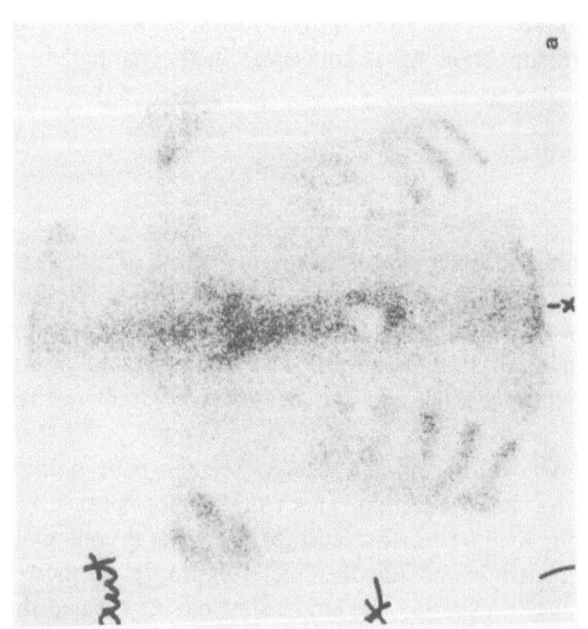

Figure 5. Two examples of artefacts. At the left hand side (a) a golden ornament, while at the right side (b) the artefact is due to a burned spot on the screen of the oscilloscope.

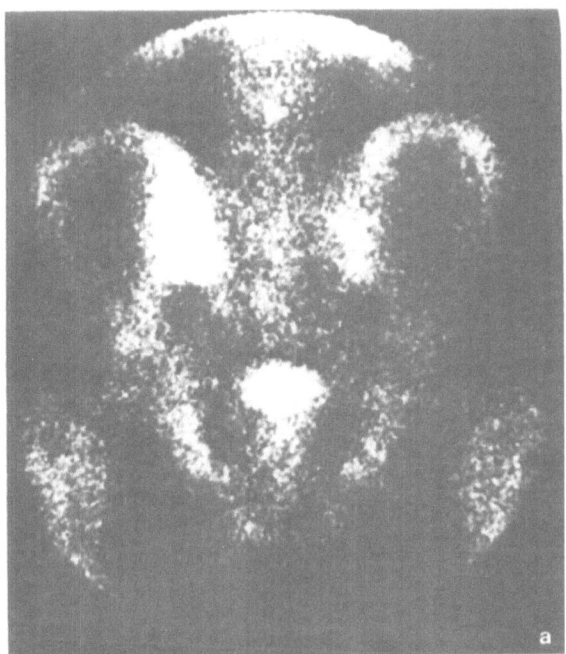

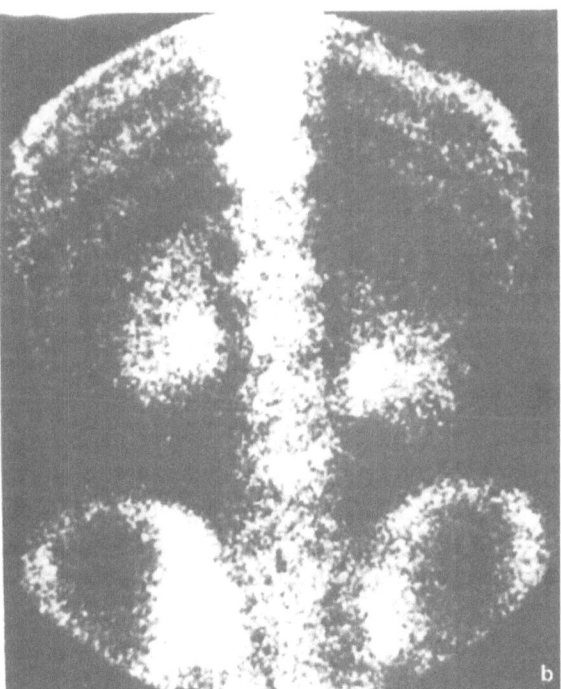

Figure 6. Bone scintigram of a patient after radiotherapy. Examination of Figure 6a could lead to the conclusion that an increased activity can be seen in the left iliac wing. Figure 6b shows the real situation of a decreased activity over the lumbar spine and right iliac wing due to the radiotherapeutic treatment.

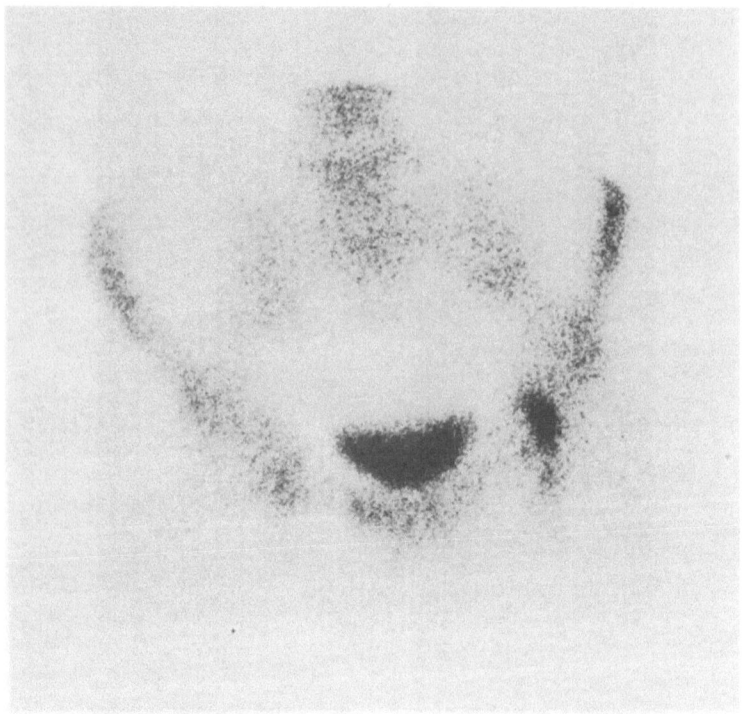

Figure 7. Bone scintigram with a hot spot over left hip region due to contamination with radioactive urine.

Labeling. In a routine laboratory occasionally labeling is not complete due to partial oxidation of Sn (II) into Sn (IV). When this occurs, unbound isotope (^{99m}Tc-pertechnetate) is found in the pharmaceutical. After injection of the preparation, this free pertechnetate will accumulate in the thyroid, salivary glands and the stomach thus obscuring part of the bone scintigram (Figure 8). For instance in the anterior and posterior view it is very difficult to distinguish between the thyroid and an abnormal cervical vertebra.

In case of large amounts of ^{99m}Tc-pertechnetate, visualization of the stomach will be present together with a poor quality bone scintigram. In a few occasions the radiopharmaceutical will be partly colloidal, due to an excess of Sn (11). This results in a distribution of radioactivity over the liver, and spleen (14).

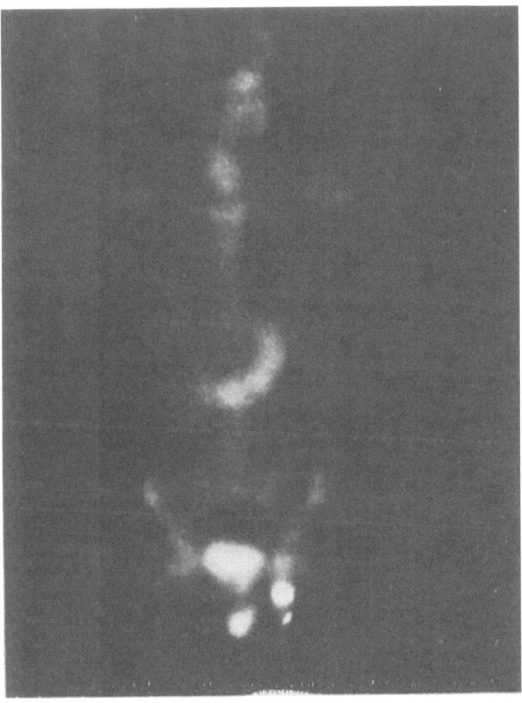

Figure 8. Bone scintigram anterior view, in which a large fraction of the radioactive material is not bound to MDP. An accumulation of the ^{99m}Tc-pertechnetate is seen over the naso-pharyngeal area, the thyroid and the stomach. Also part of the pertechnetate is excreted to the bladder. Note also the "hot spot" in the region of the left femur which is an artefact of the photographic equipment.

Soft-tissue calcification. Several investigators have reported an elevated uptake of ^{99m}Tc-phosphates in soft tissues, such as the lungs (15–17), scar tissues (18) (see Figure 9), stomach (19, 20) (see Figure 10) and myocardium (21–23). Other possible regions of increased activity are the upper legs in, for example, diabetic patients (injection site, see Figure 11) or in patients with atherosclerotic arteries. Also, patients with cerebro vascular accidents will show a deposition of radioactivity in the affected area due to deposition of calcium (Figure 12).

Radiotherapy. Directly following irradiation the bone scintigram shows an increased activity in both soft tissues and bone due to an increase of blood flow and marrow blood volume. However other mechanisms may also be responsible, such as changes in vascular permeability (24). In the second phase following radiotherapy, bone remodeling is responsible for an increased accumulation in the irradiated area. The

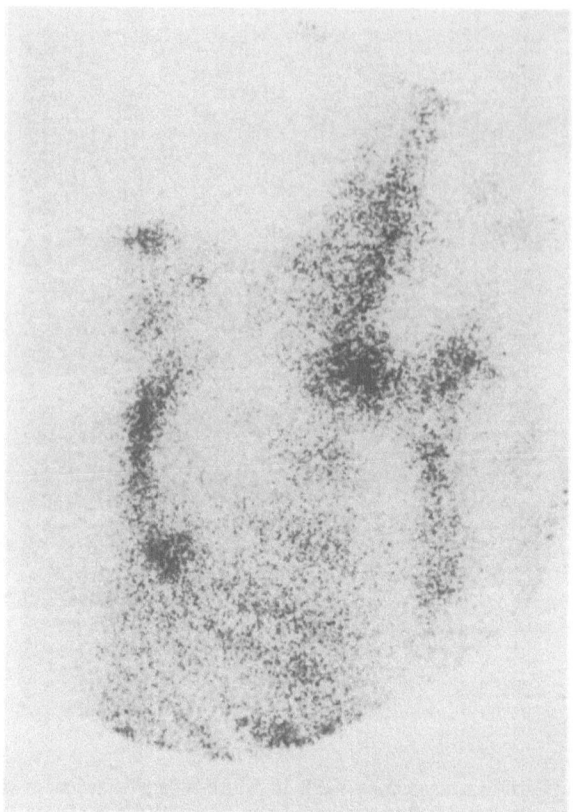

Figure 9. Bone scintigram of a patient (right oblique view), three months after thoracotomy. In the right lateral thorax an elevated activity persists due to accumulation of radioactivity in the healing ribs and in scar tissue.

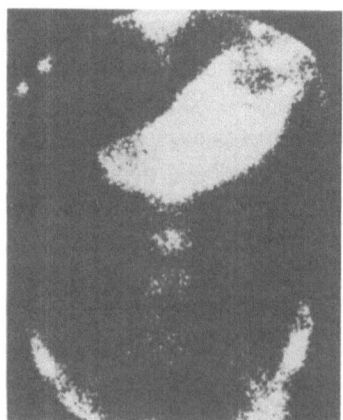

Figure 10. A patient with increased activity due to gastric calcification. No activity in the lower neck region was visible, therefore pertechnetate can be excluded.

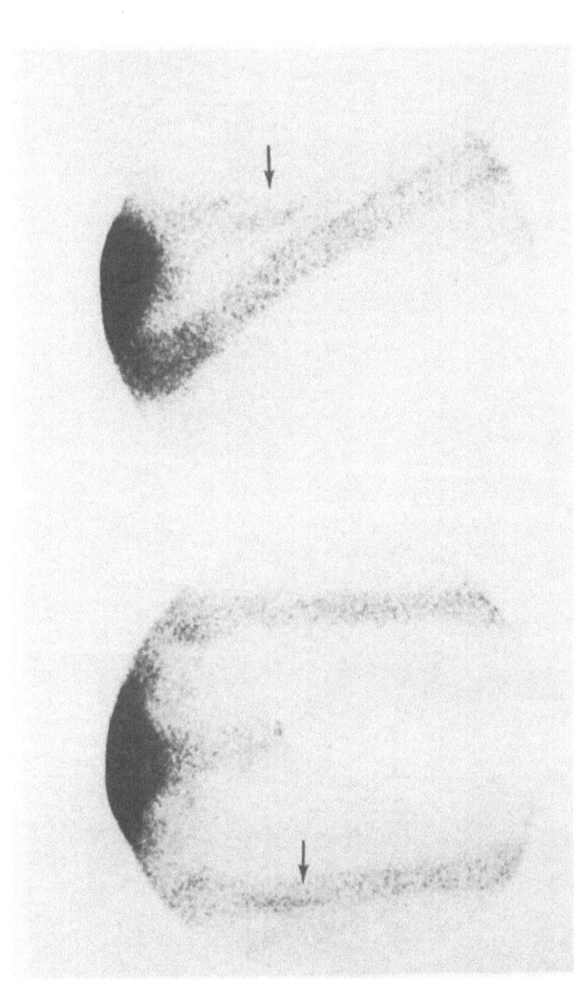

Figure 11. Increased activity in the right upper limb after treatment with several intramuscular injections. (lef-hand side, the anterior view, and at the right-hand side the right oblique view).

30

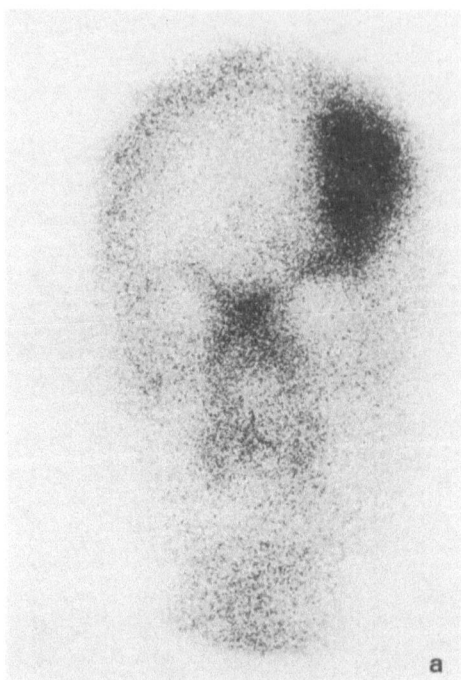

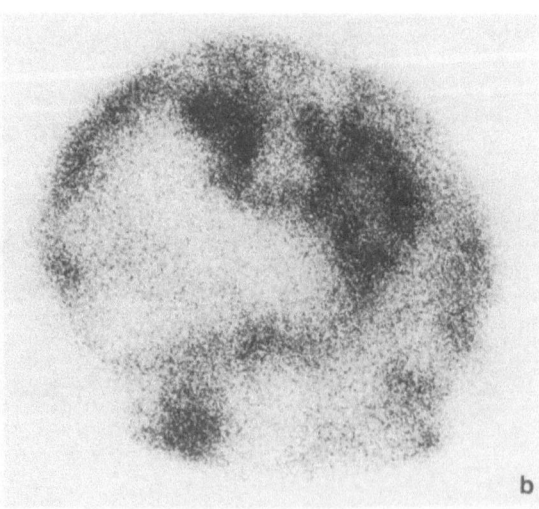

Figure 12. Bone scintigrams (anterior and right lateral views) with three-month-old cerebrovascular accident. In the anterior view a marked increase of radioactivity is noted at the left side of the skull. In the right lateral view a large area, extending from frontal to parietal, with an irregular pattern of radio-activity is shown.

soft tissues also play a role due to the possible mechanism of increased vascular permeability and an increased tissue affinity for the radiopharmaceutical, perhaps as a result of an increased calcium concentration. Cox (10) suggests an increase in cell wall permeability, which also applies to tumor cells and areas of inflammation. In the late phase following radiotherapy a depression in the blood flow ratio occurs which results in a decreased uptake of radioactivity. The time of occurrence and duration of these three post therapy phases can differ. One must, therefore, be careful not to make the mistake of diagnosing a metastasis as a postirradiated area of increased activity (Figure 13).

Infarction. Ischemic necrosis of marrow and bone is a common complication of sickle-cell disease. While signs and symptoms resemble that of osteomyelitis the treatment differs greatly. Therefore it is necessary to distinguish between these two. Osteomyelitis shows an increased activity in both early and later phases. Early images of an infarction, on

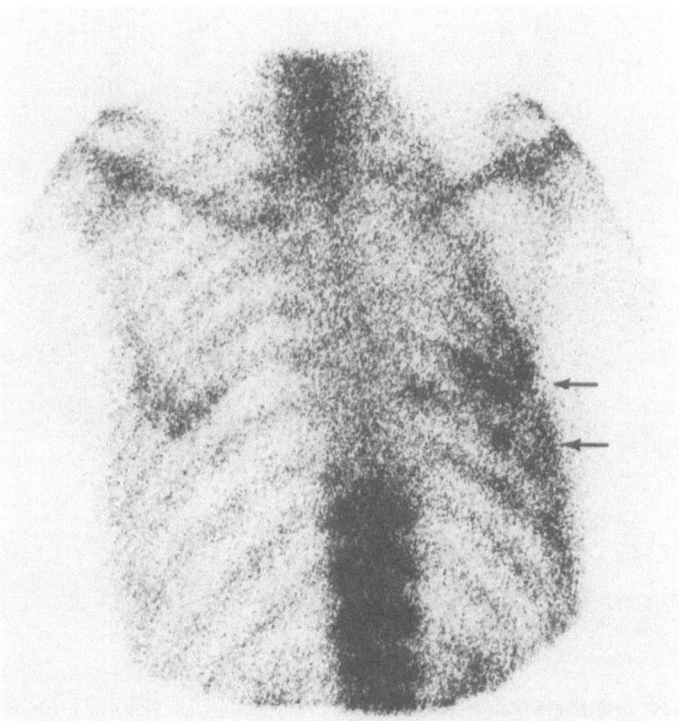

Figure 13. Bone scintigram of the thorax after radiotherapy treatment. Note the area of decreased activity (spine and ribs) together with an area of increased activity (arrow) due to metastases.

the other hand, show a normal scan, with a slightly increased activity at a later stage (Figure 14). Using high resolution collimators, or even a pinhole collimator, it is sometimes possible to identify a "cold" area of devitalized bone surrounded by an area of increased activity (due to repair).

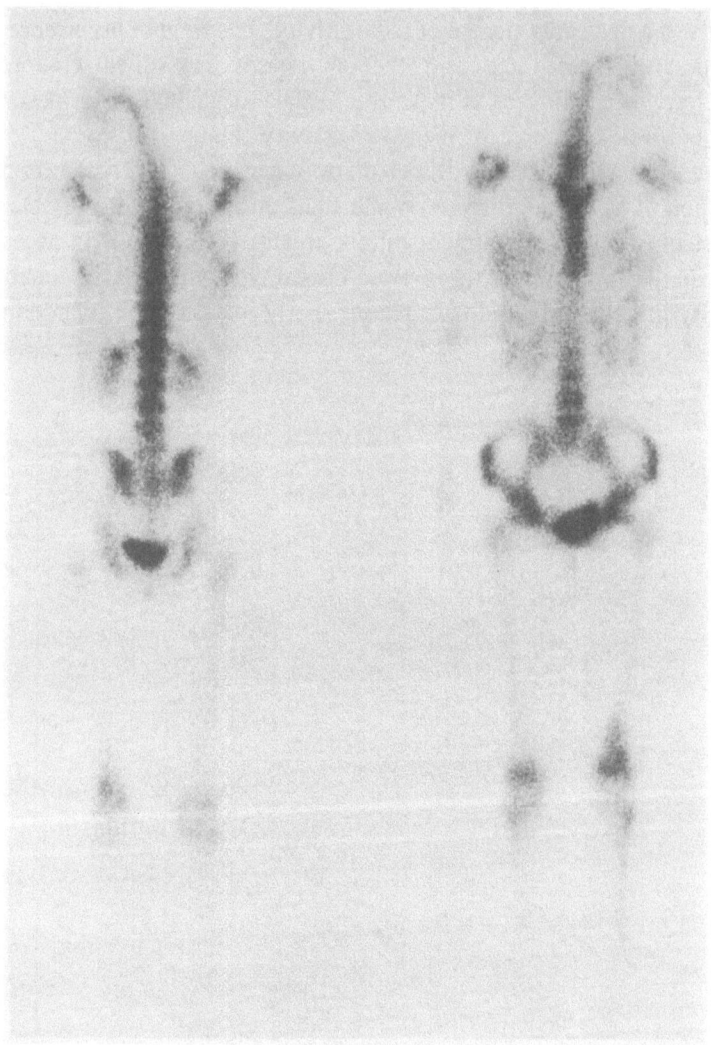

Figure 14. Late phase bone scintigram (posterior and anterior view) of a patient with a bone infarction in the distal left femur. In this scintigram only a slightly increased activity can be noted, not specific for infarction. Often a high resolution single view of the affected area will show a central core of diminished radioactivity which is characteristic for an infarction.

6. CONCLUSION

In the interpretation of bone scintigrams one must keep in mind the many factors that can lead to false negative or false positive results.

In general the problems and pitfalls of bone scintigraphy can be condensed into four main categories:

1) operator/instrumentation artefacts
2) patient variability artefacts
3) drug therapy and radiotherapy interference
4) radiopharmaceutical problems

Careful examination, considering available data and comparison with other diagnostic tools like x-ray pictures, CT-scans, ultrasound etc. can avoid many pitfalls.

REFERENCES

1. Subramanian G, McAfee JG: A new complex of ^{99m}Tc for skeletal imaging. Radiology 99:192-196, 1971.
2. Tofe AJ, Francis MD: In vitro optimization and organ distribution studies in animals with the bone scanning agent ^{99m}Tc-Sn-EHDP. J Nucl Med 13:472, 1972.
3. Yano Y, Anger HO, MacRae J, Van Dijke DC: ^{99m}Tc-labeled Sn-diphosphonate a bone scanning agent. J Nucl Med 13:480, 1972.
4. Pistenma DA, McDougall R, Kriss JP: Screening for bone metastases: are only scans necessary? JAMA 231: 46-50, 1975.
5. Rosenthall L, Kaye M: Observations on the mechanism of ^{99m}Tc-labeled phosphate complex uptake in metabolic bone disease. Seminars Nucl Med 4/1:59-67, 1976.
6. De Graaf P, Schicht IM, Pauwels EKJ, Te Velde J, de Graeff J: Bone scintigraphy in renal osteodystrophy. J Nucl Med 19:1289-1296, 1978.
7. Fogelman I, McKillop JH, Bessent RG, Boyle JT, Turner JG, Greig WR: The role of bone scanning in osteomalacia. J Nucl Med 19:245-248, 1978.
8. Handmaker H, Leonards R: The bone scan in inflammatory osseous disease. Seminars Nucl Med 6: 95-105, 1976.
9. Croft BY, Teates CD: "Lunch syndrome", a bone scanning artefact. Clin Nucl Med 3/4:137-138, 1978.
10. Cox PH: Abnormalities in skeletal uptake of ^{99m}Tc-polyphosphate complexes in areas of bone associated with tissues which have been subjected to radiation therapy. Brit J Rad 47:851-856, 1974.
11. Sorkin SJ, Horii SC, Passalaque A, Braunstein P: Decreased activity on bone scan following therapeutic radiations: a source of possible error. Clin Nucl Med 3:67-68, 1978.
12. Lutzker LG, Alavi A: Bone and marrow imaging in sickle-cell disease: diagnosis of infarction. Seminars Nucl Med 6:83-93, 1976.
13. Oppenheim BE, Cantez S: What causes lower neck uptake in bone scans? Radiology 124/3:749-752, 1977.
14. Crawford JA, Gumerman LW: Alteration of body distribution of ^{99m}Tc-pyrophosphate by radiographic contrast material. Clin Nucl Med 3:305-307, 1978.

15. Aprile C, Bernardo G, Carena M, Favino A, Robustelli della Cuna G, Strada MR, Mascherpa S: Accumulation of ^{99m}Tc-Sn-pyrophosphate in pleural effusions. Eur J Nucl Med 3:219-222, 1978.

16. De Graaf P, Schicht IM, Pauwels EKJ, Souverijn JHM, de Graeff J: Bone scintigraphy in uremic pulmonary calcification. J Nucl Med 20:201-206, 1979.

17. Curry SL: Accumulation of ^{99m}Tc-methylene diphosphonate in an adenocarcinoma of the lung. Clin Nucl Med 4:170-171, 1979.

18. Prince JR: Localization of ^{99m}Tc-diphosphonate in surgical scar. Eur J Nucl Med 4:69-71, 1979.

19. Jayabalan V, de Witt B: Gastric calcification detected in vivo by ^{99m}Tc-pyrophosphate imaging. Clin Nucl Med 3:27-29, 1978.

20. Valdez VA, Jacobstein JG, Perlmutter S, Brusman H: Metastatic calcification in lungs and stomach demonstrated on bone scan in multiple myeloma. Clin Nucl Med 4:120-121, 1979.

21. Braun SD, Lisbona R, Novales-Diaz JA, Sniderman A: Myocardial uptake of ^{99m}Tc-phosphate tracer in amyloidosis. Clin Nucl Med 4:244-245, 1979.

22. Bonte FJ, Parkey RW, Graham KD, Moore J, Stokeley EM: A new method for radionuclide imaging of myocardial infarcts. Radiology 110:473-474, 1974.

23. Parkey RW, Bonte FJ, Meyer SL, Atkins JM, Curry GL, Stokeley EM, Willerson JT: A new method for radionuclide imaging of acute myocardial infarction in humans. Circulation 50:540-546, 1975.

24. King MA, Weber DA et al: A study of irradiated bone. Part II. J Nucl Med 21:22-30, 1980.

3. RECENT DEVELOPMENTS IN BONE SCANNING

Peter J. Ell, Rohit G. Radia and Peter H. Jarritt

1. introduction

Progress in nuclear medicine is achieved through advances in radiopharmaceuticals, improvement in instrumentation design and improvement
in data processing (computer hard- and software). With the appearance
of the ^{99m}Tc-labelled phosphates (1), a major step towards finding ideal
bone seeking tracers was undertaken. The more recent modifications of
these tracers have tended to offer only minor advantages over and
above what has already been achieved, i.e., improved skeletal uptake
and somewhat faster blood clearance characteristics. Whilst computer
hard- and software is undergoing constant streamlining (more power, in
lesser space, with greater economy), instrumentation designs have
matured; this may alter the traditional way of bone scanning of the
1960's and 1970's (scanners, whole body imagers and Anger gamma
cameras). All of these techniques have relied upon conventional planar
imaging and only very recently have alternative apparatuses appeared.
The issue at stake is whether some form of tomographic imaging may
have a role to play in the investigation of the skeleton. Important and
inherent advantages occur if one is able to reconstruct data into tomograms: data interpretation is performed with the benefit of depth information, contrast resolution permits the visualization of structures previously masked and computer analysis permits the measurement of
tracer uptake within well defined sections of the organ or segment to be
investigated. In this review, we offer original data which may provide
some pointers as to future areas of application of this new approach.

2. materials and methods

We are currently investigating the performance characteristics and areas
of clinical application of a range of tomographic equipment (2, 3). All of
these techniques have in common a scintillation detector system for the

Pauwels EKJ, Schütte HE, Taconis WK, eds, Bone scintigraphy, p 35–50.
*Copyright © 1981 Martinus Nijhoff Publishers bv, The Hague/Boston/London. All rights
reserved.*

recording of emitted gamma radiation, a dedicated computer for data reconstruction into images with 3-D information (suitable algorithms are required) and are optimized for the detection of radionuclides emitting gamma photons with medium energy (single photon emission computerized tomography).

In the investigation of patients, conventional doses of standard radiopharmaceuticals were used ·(15 mCi of ^{99m}Tc-MDP- methylenediphosphonate) and imaging is performed 60 minutes after intravenous administration of the tracer. Tomograms (section scans) are usually recorded either in a single section acquisition mode (whereby each section scan or tomogram takes 4–5 minutes for data acquisition) or in a multiple section acquisition mode (with total data acquisition time of 20 minutes). In the first case, multiple detector instrumentation is used (the Cleon-710 or the Cleon-711 tomographic scanners) and in the second case, an IGE-400T rotating gamma camera is utilized linked to an Informatek-Simis-3 computer system. Whilst in the first instance, image reconstruction occurs in the transaxial plane, the rotating Anger camera and the computer system allow for immediate multiplane data reconstruction in the coronal, sagittal and transaxial planes.

In terms of patient population under scrutiny, a variety of clinical problems are under current investigation. After describing some of the section scans observed so far, details of the patients undergoing quantitation uptake measurements will be given.

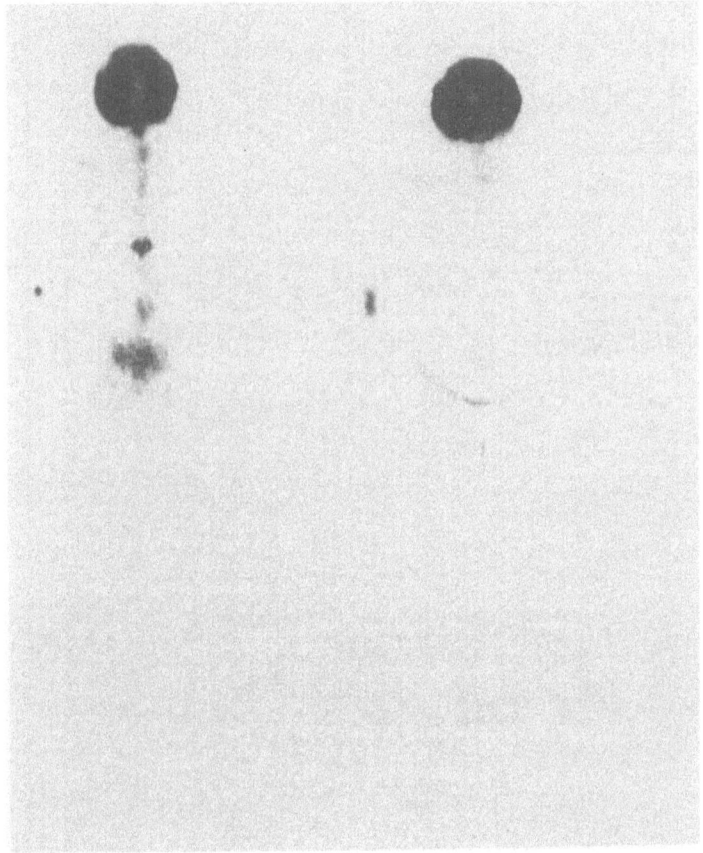

Figure 1.

Case 1. A typical whole body bone scan of a patient with advanced Paget's disease is shown (Figure 1). There is intense and abnormal tracer uptake in the entire skull, with focal uptake in several areas of the spine and sacrum. Figure 2 shows a transaxial section scan of the skull of the patient. This section scan is 13 mm thick and obtained at the level of the mid parietal bone. Note the appearance of both tables of the skull, with no or little tracer uptake in the diploe of the bone. Involvement of Paget's disease of the skull appears therefore to be non-uniform, as previously suspected.

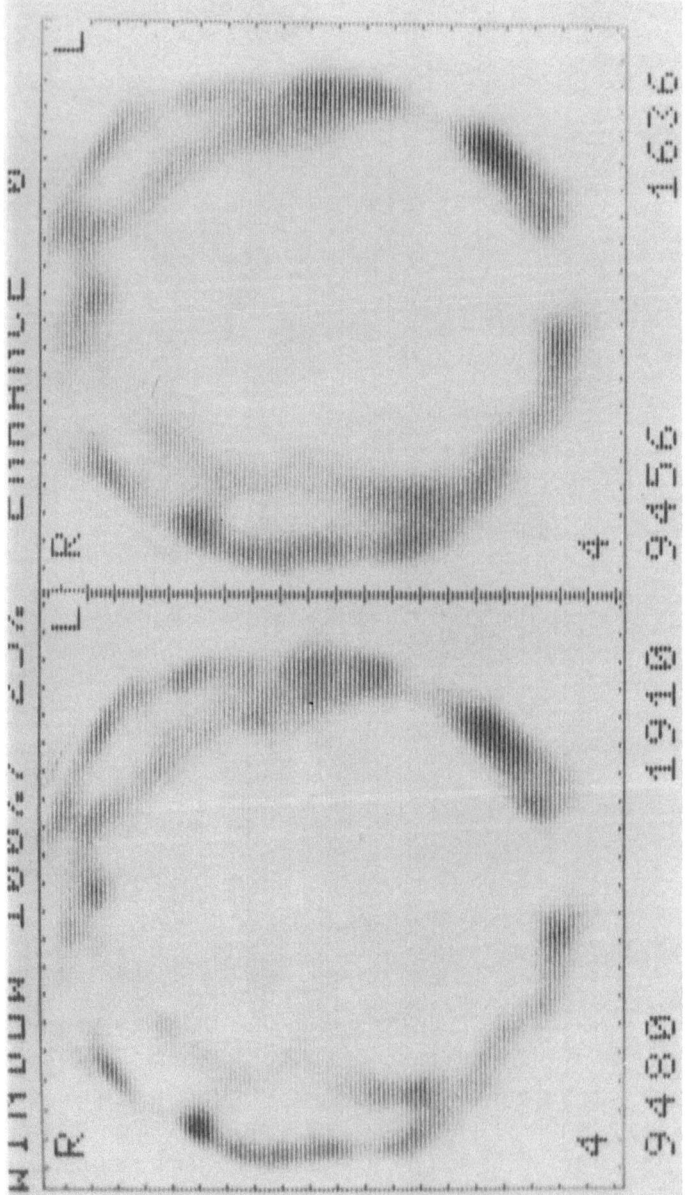

Figure 2.

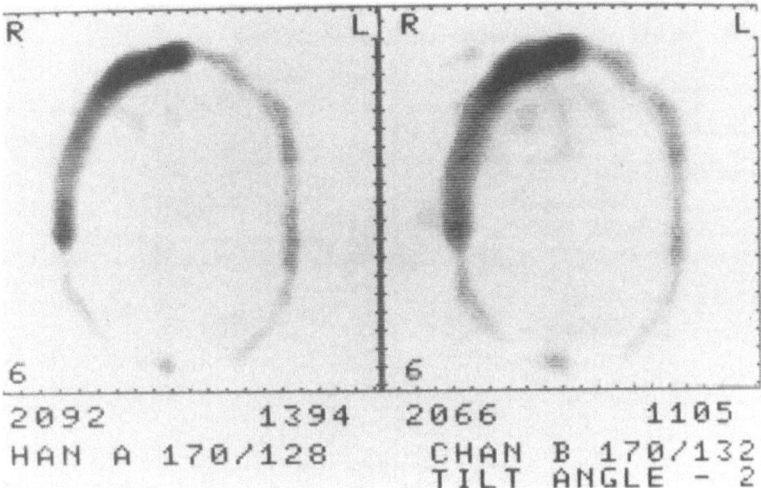

2092   1394   2066   1105
HAN A 170/128   CHAN B 170/132
                   TILT ANGLE - 2

Figure 3.

Case 2. Another case of Paget's disease is shown, and a transaxial section scan of the patient's skull (Figure 3). The section scan clearly demonstrates the ability to localize and lateralize the extent of the disease. It can be seen that it is eminently feasible to monitor more objectively possible treatment protocols or resistance to therapeutic intervention.

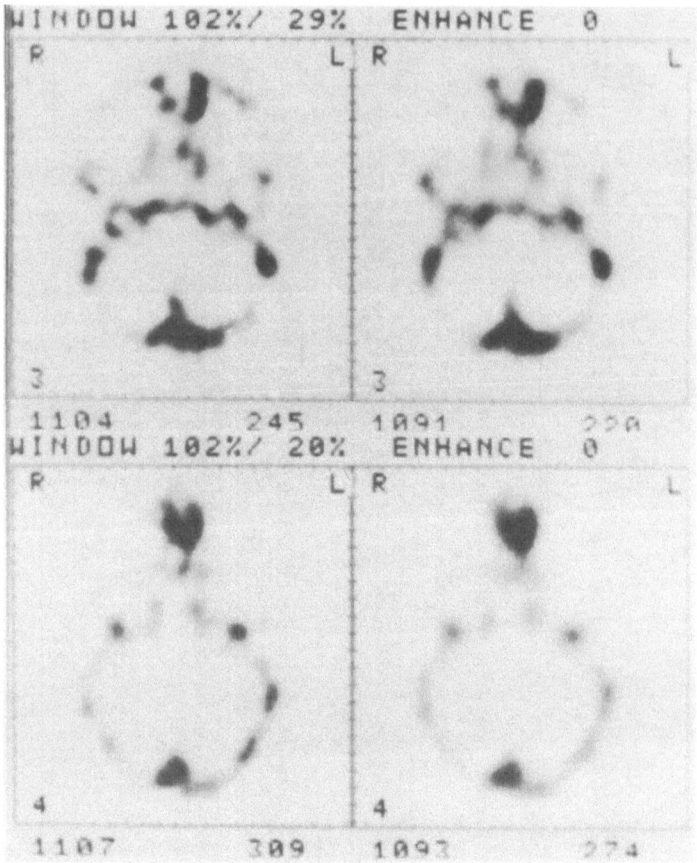

Figure 4.

Case 3. Transaxial section scans of the skull of a patient are shown (Figure 4), the underlying pathology being primary hyperparathyroidism. To note the benefit of tomography and its 3-D information. The base of the skull and its anatomy is shown to an unprecedented detail. Ordinary planar imaging is unable to display all of the structures which can be recognized on this section scan.

Case 4. A patient with carcinoma of the breast and skeletal skull secondaries. Transaxial section scans of the skull at the base (sections 2 and 3) and at the vertex (section 1) are shown (Figure 5). Multiple areas of increased and abnormal tracer uptake can be recognized, with retro-orbital deposits and secondaries in the frontal and parietal bones.

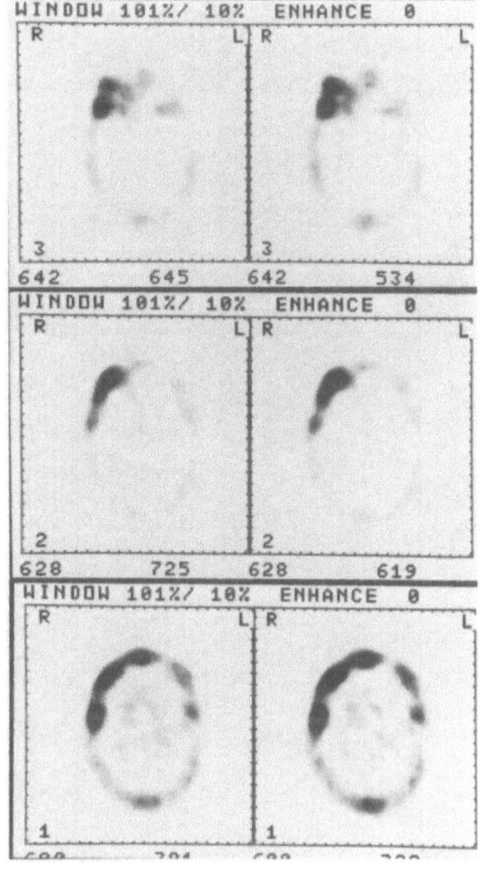

Figure 5.

→

Case 5. Figure 6 shows a conventional planar rectilinear bone scan of a patient's head and upper trunk, the standard skull x-ray and a transaxial section scan through the obvious lesion in the parietal bone. The x-ray and section scan show the complementarity of the information retrieved from these techniques. Whilst the x-ray demonstrates the destroyed and inactive bone, the section bone scan demonstrates the areas of osteoblastic activity in front and behind the main lesion, which in fact appears as a cold centre on the section scan. This information was not obtainable from the inspection of the rectilinear bone scan alone.

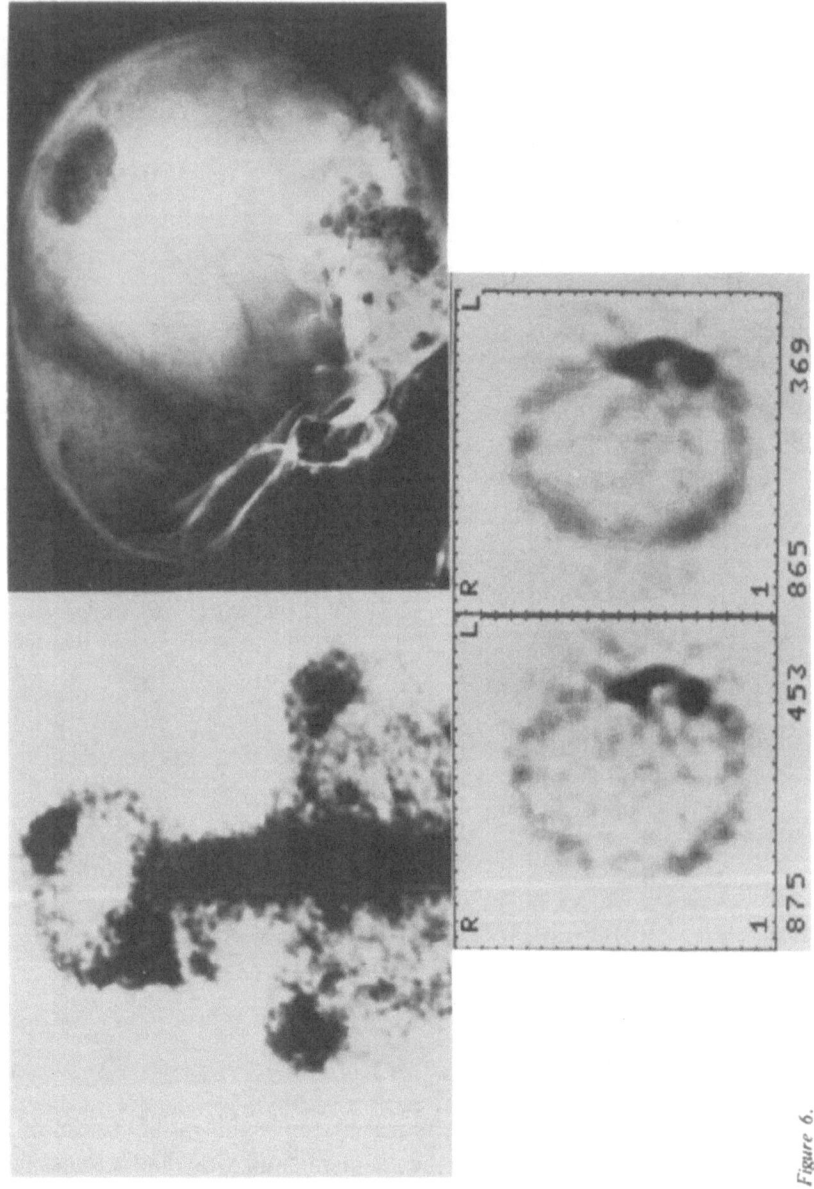

Figure 6.

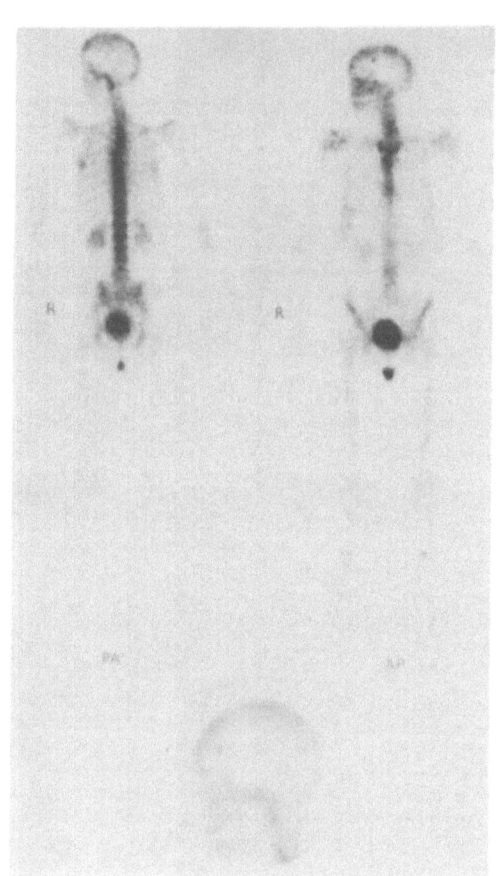

Case 6. A whole body bone scan and a detail camera view of the skull of a patient with carcinoma of the breast is shown. To note a single area of increased but focal uptake in the left frontal skull (Figure 7). The transaxial section scan through this abnormality confirms it to be sited within the bony structure of the skull (Figure 8).

Figure 7.

↓ *Figure 8.*

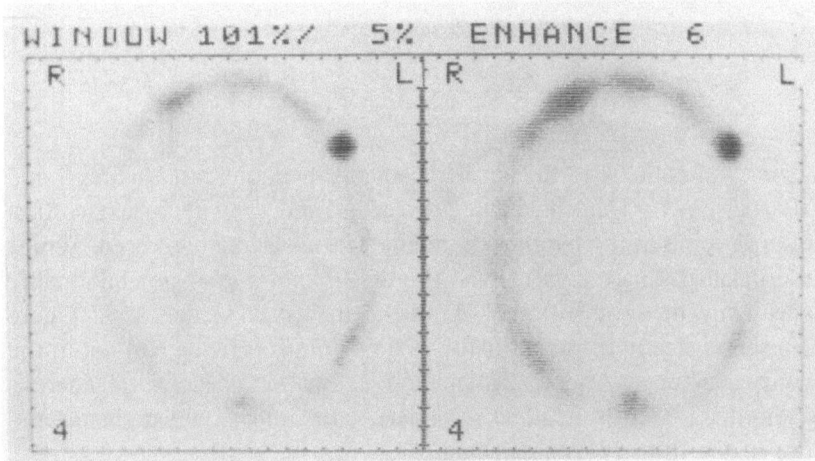

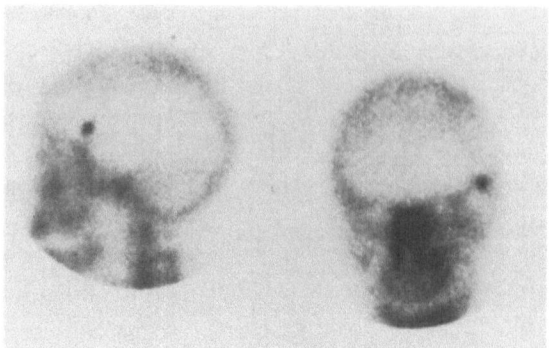

Figure 9.

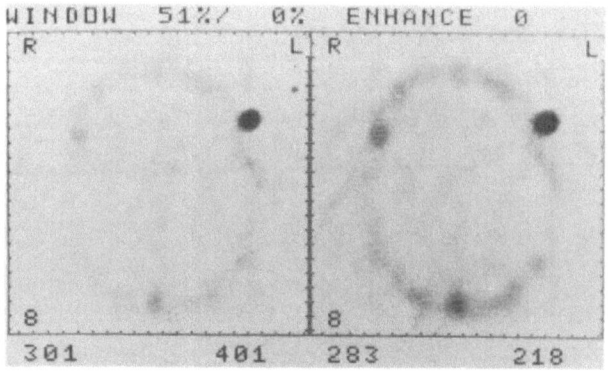

Figure 10.

Case 7. In contrast to the apparent obvious previous case, figures 9 and 10 are shown. The patient, a 56-year-old female with a juxtacortical osteosarcoma of the femur, was referred for a staging bone scan. Whilst the detailed Anger camera scan (Figure 9) shows a single abnormality apparently in the left frontal skull, the transaxial section scan (Figure 10) shows clearly the abnormality to lie within soft tissue and not in the bony structures. After palpation and extirpation, histological analysis showed a 2.4 mm soft tissue secondary with similar cellular characteristics of the primary osteosarcoma.

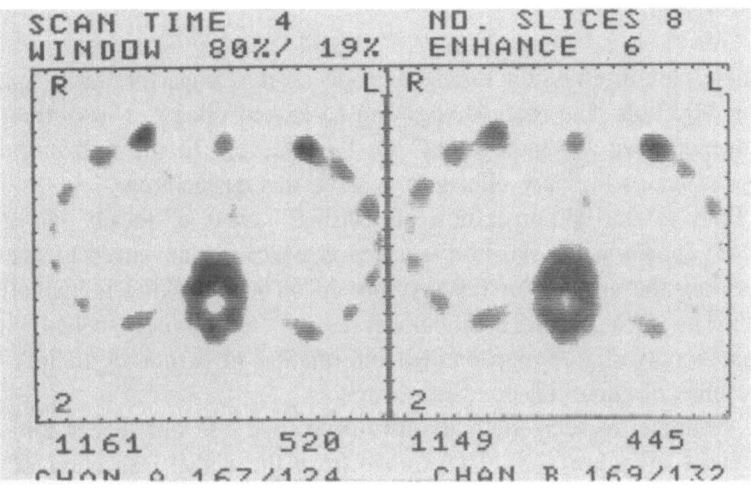

Figure 11.

Case 8. A transaxial section scan of the chest of a young patient referred for staging of his osteosarcoma is shown (Figure 11). Note the distribution of the tracer in the growing skeleton (ribs in particular) with excellent definition of the spinal canal. This information is seen for the first time and is unobtainable from a conventional and planar bone scan.

Case 9. A transaxial section scan of a femur (Figure 12). To note a zoomed view on the left, with the standard section scan on the right.

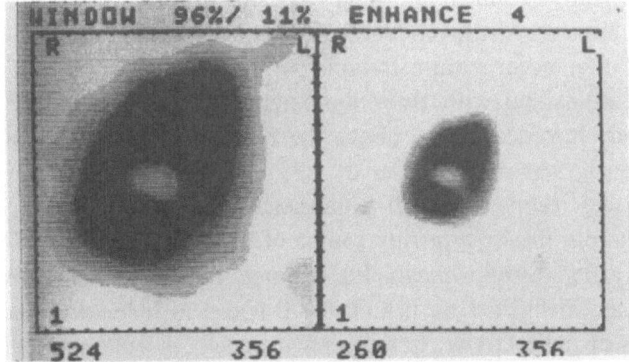

Figure 12.

2.1. *Tracer uptake*

Single photon emission tomography does offer scope for tracer uptake quantification. The methodology can be looked upon as a way through which in vivo autoradiography can be achieved. In the following, we report our preliminary efforts to achieve this desideratum.

Prior to the demonstration of "visible" areas of focally increased tracer uptake in the skeleton (such as is typical for advanced metastatic disease), the analysis of the distribution of bone seeking radiopharmaceuticals such as those in current use (^{99m}technetium-labelled phosphates) may still contain enough information to permit to identify the presence of abnormal bone turnover.

A number of such methods have been tried out and appeared in the relevant literature (4, 5). They range from the visual inspection of the patterns of phosphate distribution in the whole body bone scan to the measurement of a variety of indices. These include the amount of this type of radiopharmaceutical retained in the body at 24 hours as measured via whole body counting, the calculation of a variety of bone to soft tissue ratios, and so on. Most of these studies have been exclusively directed towards the investigation of metabolic bone disease and so far, none has utilized the tomographic scanning approach.

The aim of the pilot study which we are describing was to utilize a computerized tomographic emission scanner (Cleon-710) and establish the feasibility of defining ranges of tracer uptake in the skull of a normal population, to express this tracer uptake in terms of µCi of ^{99m}Tc-MDP per ml of active skull volume and to apply the established normal ranges to the investigation of a diseased population.

The following procedure was adopted: for scanning purposes, the Cleon-710 brain scanner with a FWHM of 9 mm and 3.6 K cps/µCi/ml as the sensitivity index for ^{99m}Tc was utilized. 15 mCi of ^{99m}Tc-MDP were administered intravenously and imaging was commenced 60 to 90 minutes after tracer administration. For each section scan, four minutes of data acquisition with three tomograms recorded per study. Section scans were recorded 2.5 cm above the External Acustical Meatus plane, slice spacing was of the order of 1.25 cm. Slice thickness was 1.3 cm, with images reconstructed in a transaxial plane.

A phantom (basically a ring source of uniform activity of ^{99m}Tc) was used to calibrate the tomographic scanner. Linearity of this instrumentation was established by testing its response to increasing and known amounts of radioactivity. It was shown that for a wide range of activity concentrations (between 0.05 µCi/ml to 5 µCi/ml), the tomographic scanner responded in a linear fashion. A basic assumption was made (which holds for non-focal disease in the skull) and that is that the ring phantom used actually simulates the shape and activity distribution within the skull. Three methods were used in the calculation of μCi/ml of ^{99m}Tc-MDP skull uptake:

Method A consisting of ring source calibration, no background subtraction and a maximum pixel count;

Method B consisting of ring source calibration, 25% background subtraction and an average pixel count;

Method C consisting of ring source calibration, variable background subtraction and an average pixel count.

For method A, and in 40 normal volunteers, a mean value of 0.11 μCi/ml for ^{99m}Tc-MDP uptake was obtained (range 0.08–0.14). For method B, and in 11 normal volunteers, a mean value of 0.06μCi/ml for ^{99m}Tc-MDP uptake was obtained (range 0.05–0.07). For method C, and in 11 normal volunteers, a mean value of 0.03 μCi/ml for ^{99m}Tc-MDP uptake was obtained (range 0.02–0.04).

It is interesting to note that the normal values recorded in this population showed rather narrow ranges. So far, method B, wich we feel is at present the most appropriate, was utilized for the calculation of ^{99m}Tc-MDP skull tracer uptake values in a series of diseased individuals. 17 patients with skeletal deposits other than in the skull were investigated, 5 patients with Paget's disease, 4 patients with osteomalacia, 3 patients post parathyroidectomy, 1 patient with primary hyperparathyroidism and 1 patient with thyrotoxicosis were investigated.

A preliminary study is in progress whereby patients with osteomalacia are being monitored with a base line study and then at repeated intervals, on commencement of treatment. Figures 13 and 14 summarize the initial patient data.

The data shows quite clearly the feasibility of the method of tracer quantification and its ability to distinguish a normal from an abnormal population. There is an interesting pointer in the data which stems from patients suffering from skeletal metastases other than in the skull. Even this group of patients show a much higher tracer uptake than the normal ranges calculated (the horizontal bar in the graphs indicates the normal range). One can speculate on the possible reasons for this, and work is in progress to establish the role of substances such as PTH. It might just be that if this trend were to continue in a larger group of patients, that earlier recognition of bony secondaries might be feasible prior to their detection as areas of focal increased tracer deposition ("hot spots").

48

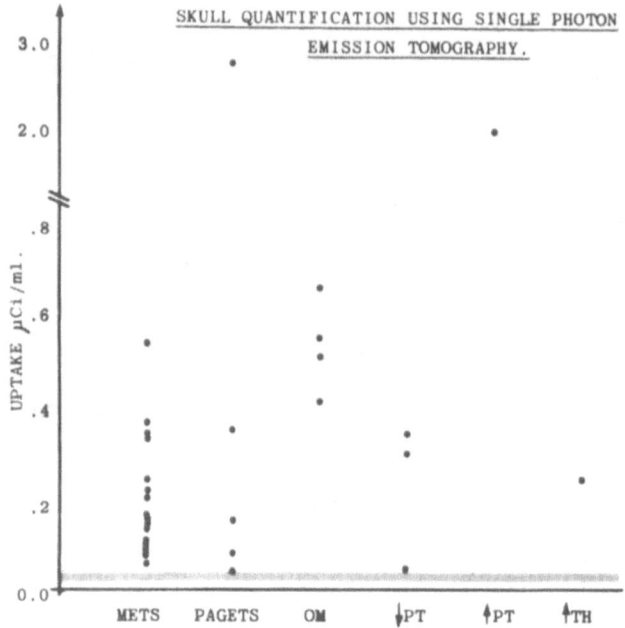

Figure 13. Tracer (^{99m}Tc-MDP) uptake values in normals and abnormal patients.

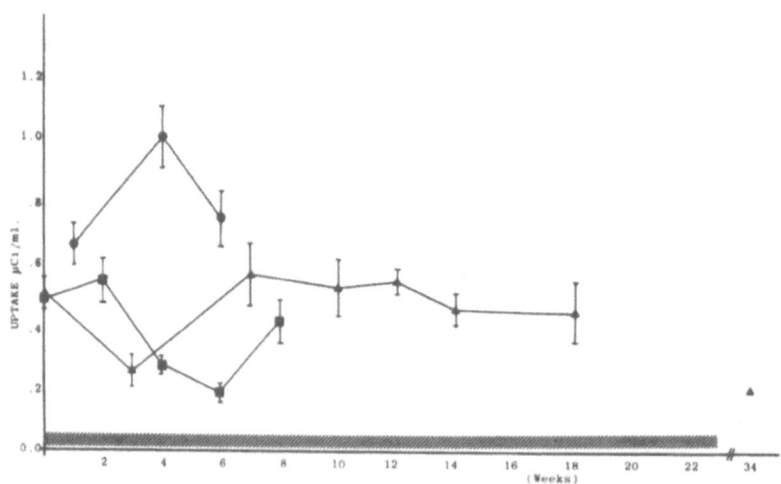

Figure 14. Follow-up study in 3 patients with osteomalacia.

The osteomalacia group of patients were all classical clinical cases of this condition, due to dietary vitamin D deficiency. Reduced serum calcium and phosphate levels, raised serum alkaline phosphatase and parathyroid hormone levels were seen. As predicted for patients with secondary hyperparathyroidism, raised ^{99m}Tc-MDP skull uptake values were observed.

In the serial evaluation of patients with osteomalacia during therapy with 1,25, dihydroxycholecalciferol, there was initial reduction of tracer uptake in the skull, followed by a increase to nearly pretreatment levels and a later slow tapering of these values. Elevated uptake levels were still present six months after commencement of treatment. One might speculate that one of the possible mechanisms involved in the initial reduction of tracer uptake in the skull is that the normalization of serum calcium leads to a flattening of the stimulus to hyperparathyroidism, resulting in a temporary state of hypoparathyroidism.

Three patients with a laryngopharyngectomy have been studied. These patients are on supplements of vitamin D_3, calcium and thyroxine. The two patients who show wide fluctuations in serum biochemistry and poor clinical control also show elevated tracer uptake. The third patient has maintained near normal serum biochemistry on supplements and has normal skull tracer uptake as measured by our techniques.

3. CONCLUSION

It is clear that this data is rather exciting. It is also apparent that quantification of tracer uptake in the skeleton appears to open new avenues for thought and possibly original fields for the application of bone scanning techniques to clinical problems. Whether or not a tomographic approach is indispensable for these type of measurements and assessments remains to be seen. Nevertheless, emission tomography is the only technique which permits the evaluation of tracer uptake in terms of unit of tracer per unit of volume or weight of the organ or system under study. It is this unique capability (coupled with the display of 3-D images) which permits one to hope in its future potential. With almost ideal tracers, such as the ^{99m}Tc labelled phosphates, very small lesions can be detected and followed. The smallest measured lesion detected with the tomograpic techniques was of the order of 2.4 mm. Normal ranges of tracer uptake have been measured in an already significant normal population (n = 40) and shown to be reproducible and with a rather narrow range of values. One striking feature is the indication of the great difference in tracer uptake values found in the skull be the time some of these patients are referred for investigation. There is therefore a clearcut normal/abnormal gradient which can be explored. Further studies are in progress in order to elucidate some of the pathophysiological issues raised during this feasibility trial.

REFERENCES

1. Subramanian G, McAfee JG: A new complex of ^{99m}Tc for skeletal imaging. Radiology 99:192-196, 1971.
2. Jarritt PH, Ell PJ, Myers MJ, Brown NJG, Deacon JM: A new transverse section brain imager for single gamma emitters. J Nucl Med 20 (4):319-327, 1979.
3. Jarritt PH, Ell PJ: A new emission tomographic body scanner. Nuclear Medicine Communications 1 (2):94-101, 1980.
4. Fogelman I, Bessent RG, Turner JG, Citrin DL, Boyle IT, Greig WR: The use of whole body retention of ^{99m}Tc-diphosponate in the diagnosis of metabolic bone disease. J Nucl Med 19:270-275, 1978.
5. Rosenthall L, Lisbona R: Role of radionuclide imaging in benign bone and joint diseases of orthopaedic interest. In: Nuclear medicine annual, Freeman LM, Weissmann H (eds), New York, Raven Press, 1980, no 1, p 267-301.

PART II

BONE SCINTIGRAPHY
IN BENIGN DISEASE

4. SCINTIGRAPHY IN INFLAMMATORY OSSEOUS DISEASE

PAUL B. HOFFER and ROBERT PRINCENTHAL

Anatomical distribution
Diagnosis of osteomyelitis
Diagnostic approach
Interpretation of negative results

1. INTRODUCTION

Osteomyelitis and joint infections are serious diseases which occur most frequently in children and young adults. They are also seen in individuals with diathesis toward infection due to underlying systemic disease, e.g. diabetes. In children and young adults the source of infection is usually hematogenous; involvement from adjacent soft tissue infections is more frequent in adults, especially diabetics.

Joint infections are usually treated by drainage, if possible, followed by a 3–4 week course of appropriate antibiotic therapy (1, 2). Treatment of osteomyelitis requires long-term (4–6 weeks) antibiotic therapy (3). The antibiotic is usually administered intravenously for the entire 6-week course of therapy, although modified regimens of intravenous (2 weeks) followed by oral (4 weeks) treatment may be adequate in acute lesions (4).

Attitudes toward local drainage vary from institution to institution, some preferring drainage of radiographically evident abscesses only, while others consider localizing symptoms in the face of a clinical diagnosis as adequate indication.

2. ANATOMICAL DISTRIBUTION

Osteomyelitis occurs most commonly in the metaphyseal region of long bones in children and adjacent to sites of chronic soft tissue ulcerations in adults. While the epiphyseal plate usually acts as a barrier to spread of infection into adjacent joint areas in older children, it does not provide this protection in infants (up to 1 year old) or adults. Therefore

Pauwels EKJ, Schütte HE, Taconis WK, eds, Bone scintigraphy, p 53–58.

osteomyelitis in infants and adults will frequently involve adjacent joints (3). Also there are increasing numbers of cases of osteomyelitis in children involving the spine, skull, pelvis and small bones of the extremities (5, 6, 7, 8, 9).

3. DIAGNOSIS OF OSTEOMYELITIS

Radiographic diagnosis of osteomyelitis in the acute phase lacks sensitivity. While subtle radiographic changes may be detectable as early as the third day following onset of symptoms (10), most patients have neither radiographic changes (11) nor radiographic signs which can be distinguished from other chronic disease. The later problem is especially significant in diabetics. The use of tomography or CT scanning may improve the sensitivity, especially in areas such as the spine (12, 13).

Bone scanning with ^{99m}Tc phosphate compounds has been heralded as a highly sensitive method of early diagnosis of both osteomyelitis and joint infection. A review of numerous large series reveals an overall sensitivity of 92% (244/264) and a specificity of 95% (258/272) for detection of osteomyelitis in patients with clinical symptoms (5–8, 11–13, 15–22).

However numerous cautions have recently been expressed regarding the use of this technique. In a review of bone imaging in infants and children, Harcke quotes Ash as reporting a high incidence of false-negative bone scans for osteomyelitis in neonates (23). It is possible, though unproven, that this may relate to the difference in metaphyseal blood supply in infants up to 1 year of age as compared to older children (3).

Handmaker and Leonards emphasize that osteomyelitis may present as a " cold " defect on bone scan and that joint infections in children are often not detectable on bone scan during the acute phase (24). Numerous case reports emphasize that osteomyelitis in older children may also present initially without bone scan changes (6, 7, 12, 15–17, 22, 25).

Gilday and associates (7) have advocated the routine use of an early "blood pool" phase image as well as a later bone phase image to distinguish cellulitis from true osteomyelitis. Areas of cellulitis are positive on the early image yet show normal bone uptake on later images. Osteomyelitis is associated with increased activity on the late image. Handmaker has suggested that bone infarcts can be distinguished from osteomyelitis by their scan appearance (17), infarcts showing normal or only slightly increased uptake. We have had less success distinguishing between infarct and abscess. More recently numerous investigators have

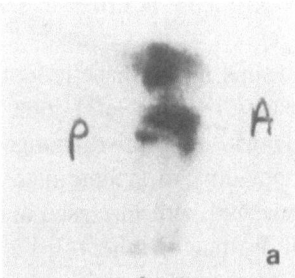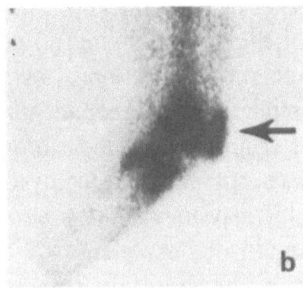

Figure 1. Bone scan performed with ^{99m}Tc MDP (A, lateral view) demonstrates no abnormality in this young patient with right knee pain and swelling. A gallium-67 citrate scan performed immediately after (B, 24-hour post-injection image, lateral view shown) demonstrates increased activity in the right patella. Osteomyelitis of the right patella was surgically confirmed.

advocated the use of the ^{67}Ga scan for early detection of osteomyelitis. The ^{67}Ga scan is usually positive even when the bone scan is normal.

Our experience with use of the bone scan for detection of osteomyelitis, septic disc infections or septic arthritis has yielded mixed results (22). While the bone scan is usually positive in acute osteomyelitis, only about 50% of such lesions are "obvious". An additional 30% of cases demonstrate either subtle findings or present a scan image indistinguishable from a septic arthritis, i.e. diffuse uptake in all bone surrounding the articular cartilage. The remaining 20% of cases present no evidence of increased uptake on the initial bone scan! (See Figure 1.) The reason for this high incidence of false-negative scans is unclear. Only two of the four patients in this group were neonates.

The etiology of these false negative bone scans may be of significance as it relates to misdiagnosis and potential delay in or failure to institute appropriate therapy. Localization of ^{99m}Tc phosphate compounds in bone is, to a large measure, a function of bone blood flow. Therefore the absence of increased radionuclide uptake at the site of bone infection suggests impairement of hyperemic response to the infection. Garnett and associates, in their report of a bone scan negative case of osteomyelitis suggest that increased local pressure and/or small vessel thrombosis may be responsible for the prevention of a hyperemic response (8). It is highly probable that such cases, because of the compromised blood supply in the region of the lesion, may be the most susceptible to recurrence and require the most aggressive long term treatment.

While we have not reported our experience with joint infections, it parallels that of bone infection, most cases being positive on scan but a significant minority showing no changes.

The problem of detection of osteomyelitis in the diabetic foot is even more complicated. These patients frequently have local joint disease. Moreover neuropathic osteoarthropathy with resorptive changes in the tarsal bones can mimic osteomyelitis not only in symptomatology and radiographic appearance but is also associated with increased activity on bone scan. In our experience, as well as that of others (3, 13, 18), the ^{67}Ga scan is almost always positive in osteomyelitis and joint infection, even in those cases in which bone scan is normal.

Also, the extent of gallium uptake is a useful guide in determining the presence or absence of active disease when the bone scan is positive. When the bone scan changes are related to chronic inactive disease or noninfectious etiology, the gallium scan is rarely more than faintly positive. If, however an active inflammatory process is present, the gallium scan will show markedly increased uptake. The only situation in which this dictum does not hold true is when tumor is present, in which case both the bone and gallium scans will show increased uptake. The chief difficulty in use of the gallium scan for diagnosis of bone and joint infections is distinguishing soft tissue inflammation from bone involvement.

4. DIAGNOSTIC APPROACH

Our current approach to the diagnosis of suspected bone and joint infection is to obtain initial radiographs. Assuming the radiographs are not diagnostic, we then proceed to a ^{99m}Tc phosphate bone scan. We no longer perform an initial blood pool image since we have not found the diagnosis of cellulitis by this method to be clinically useful. Our rational behind performing the bone scan in spite of its limitations is as follows: It is fast and inexpensive; the radiopharmaceutical is readily available and, when positive, the scan confirms the diagnosis. The bone scan will be positive in about 80%–90% of cases of osteomyelitis. Even in situations in which we know the scan will be abnormal, e.g. the diabetic foot, it serves as a useful comparative study.

5. INTERPRETATION OF NEGATIVE RESULTS

If the bone scan is negative and infection is strongly suspected clinically or if the bone scan is positive but underlying chronic noninflammatory disease is present, we proceed to a gallium scan. We will never report a negative bone scan as having "ruled out" osteomyelitis or joint infection. If the gallium scan is clearly positive and obviously involves bone, we will diagnose osteomyelitis even if the bone scan is normal. If no increased gallium uptake is observed we feel that an acute inflammatory process is unlikely, even if the bone scan is positive. Confusion arises when gallium uptake in inflammed soft tissues surrounding a bone or joint makes determination of involvement of specific bone or joint structures impossible. In such cases we will usually suggest a repeat study once the local soft tissue inflammatory process has been controlled with antibiotics.

We find this approach is highly sensitive and specific in diagnosing bone and joint infections in children and most adults. While our results in diagnosis of pedal osteomyelitis in diabetics are less accurate, the technique is still frequently useful.

One final caveat should be observed. In performing bone scans and gallium scans in children and young adults, we always prefer to survey all bones and joints. We occasionally find multiple sites of involvement in patients who present initially with symptoms referable to only one location.

The bone scan is not useful in following the progress of antibiotic therapy since it may remain positive long after the infection has resolved. We prefer the gallium scan for monitoring therapy (if clinically indicated) and in detection of suspected recurrence of disease.

REFERENCES

1. Blockey NJ, Watson JT: Acute osteomyelitis in children. J Bone Joint Surg 52(B):77-87, 1970.
2. Mollan RA, Piggot J: Acute osteomyelitis in children. J Bone Joint Surg 59(B):2-7, 1977.
3. Waldvogel FA, Medoff G, Swartz Mn: Osteomyelitis: a review of clinical features, therapeutic consideration and unusual aspects. N Engl J Med 287:198-206, 260-266, 316-322.
4. Prober CG, Yeager AS: Use of the serum bactericidal titer to assess the adaquacy of oral antibiotic therapy in the treatment of acute hematogenous osteomyelitis. J Pediatrics 95:131-135, 1979.
5. Ailsby RL, Staheli LT: Pyogenic infections of the sacroiliac joint in children. Clin Orthopedics and Related Res 100:96-100, 1974.
6. Duszynski D, Kuhn JP, Afshani E, Riddles Berger, MM: Early radionuclide diagnosis of acute osteomyelitis. Radiology 117:337-340, 1975.
7. Gilday DL, Paul DJ, Paterson J: diagnosis of osteomyelitis in children by combined blood pool and bone imaging. Radiology 117:311-335, 1975.
8. Majd M: Radionuclide imaging in early detection of childhood osteomyelitis and its differentiation from cellulitis and bone infarction. Annals Radiology 20:9-18, 1977.

58

9. Nixon G: Hematogenous osteomyelitis of metaphyseal-equivolent locations. Am J Roentgenol 130:123-129, 1978.
10. Capitanio M, Kirkpatrick A: Early roentgen observations in acute osteomyelitis. Am J Roentgenol 108:488-496, 1978.
11. Treves S, Khettry J, Broker FH, Wilkinson RH, Watts H: Osteomyelitis: early scintigraphic detection in children. Pediatrics 57:173-185, 1976.
12. Bolivar R, Kohn S, Pickering LK: Vertebral osteomyelitis in children: a report of 4 cases. Pediatrics 62:549-553, 1978.
13. Kuhn JP, Berger PE: Computed tomographic diagnosis of osteomyelitis. Radiology 130:503-506, 1979.
14. Epremian BE, Perez LA: Imaging strategy in osteomyelitis. Clin Nucl Med 2:218-220, 1977.
15. Garnet ES, Cockshott WP, Jacobs J: Classical acute osteomyelitis with a negative bone scan. Br J Radiol 50:No 598, 757-760, 1977.
16. Gelfand MJ, Silberstain EB: Radionuclide imaging: Use in diagnosis of osteomyelitis in children. JAMA 237:245-247, 1977.
17. Handmaker H, Giommona ST: The 'Hot-Joint' – increased diagnostic accuracy using combined ^{99m}Tc and ^{67}Ga-citrate imaging in pediatrics. J Nucl Med 17:554 (AB), 1976.
18. Kucera H, Mastbeck A, Anamm E: The value of scintigraphy for the early detection of osteomyelitis. Paediats Paedol (German) 13:153-158, 1978.
19. Letts RM, Afifi A, Sutherland JB: Technetium bone scanning as an aid in the diagnosis of atypical acute osteomyelitis. Surg Gyn Ob 140:899-902, 1975.
20. Lisbona R, Rosenthall L: Observations on the sequential use of 99mTechnetium and 67-Ga imaging in osteomyelitis, cellulitis, and septic arthritis. Radiology 123:123-129, 1977.
21. McKay WJ, Andrews JT, Thomas DP: The value of bone scan in early diagnosis of infective skeletal pathology. Australasian Radiology 22:165-169, 1978.
22. Sullivan D, Rosenfield NS, Ogden J, Gottschalk A: Problems in the scintigraphic detection of osteomyelitis in children. Radiology 135: 731-736, 1980.
23. Harcke TH: Bone imaging in infants and children: a review. J Nucl Med 19: 324-329, 1978.
24. Handmaker H, Leonards R: Bone scan in inflammatory osseous disease. Semin Nucl Med 6:95-105, 1976.
25. Teates CD, Williamson RJ: "Hot and cold" bone lesion in acute osteomyelitis. Am J Roentgenol 129:517-518, 1977.

5. FRACTURES AND BENIGN BONE TUMOURS

MALCOLM V. MERRICK

1. FRACTURE

1.1. *Mechanisms*

The sequence of histological changes which may be observed following fracture is well documented. There is a corresponding changing pattern of uptake of radioactive bone-seeking isotopes. This pattern is essentially similar for all radiopharmaceuticals which have been studied (1–3). The clearance of ^{18}F from soft tissues is faster than that of the technetium labelled complexes. Apart from this there are no important differences between them (4).

Immediately after fracture, the defect between the broken ends of the bone is filled by extravasated blood and inflammatory exudate. Imaging with radioisotopes at this time shows only diffusely increased uptake, mainly due to the soft tissue hyperaemia. Large avascular regions, for example blood clots or bone which has lost its blood supply, may be identified as photon-deficient areas within the traumatised site. The extent and duration of this depends upon many factors, but especially the mechanism of injury, the amount of bone which has been deprived of its blood supply and the severity of the trauma. In the adult the most important blood supply to most long bones comes via the periosteum. Separation from periosteum is therefore the commonest cause of avascularity.

Granulation tissue starts to form immediately and is easily recognisable within 24 hours of injury. Simultaneously it begins to differentiate

Pauwels EKJ, Schütte HE, Taconis WK, eds, Bone scintigraphy, p 59–80.
Copyright © 1981 Martinus Nijhoff Publishers bv, The Hague/Boston/London. All rights reserved.

into callus. This is associated with the start of reabsorption of necrotic and damaged tissue, and the beginning of new bone formation in the healty bone on both sides of the fracture line. Granulation tissue is associated with a local increase in blood flow and progressive augmentation of the capillary surface area available for exchange (5, 6). Imaging at this time therefore shows distinct areas of increased uptake on either side of the fracture line, separated by a photon-deficient area (7). The clarity with which the two areas may be distinguished depends on their separation and on the available resolution of the imaging device. Although increased bone uptake (as distinct from soft tissue uptake) is found within a few hours of injury (8), it may be concealed by the soft tissue hyperaemia for several days.

As healing progresses, devitalised tissue is removed from both sides of the fracture line, and new osteoid is laid down and calcified. The two areas of increased bone turnover, and therefore increased isotope uptake, progressively approach each other and eventually coalesce, preceeding radiological evidence of union by some weeks. This, however, may reflect only the difference in resolution between radiological and radioisotope imaging devices. Increased uptake may persist for a considerable time after radiological union is apparently complete (9).

1.2. *Applications*

This pattern is seen clearly in experimental animals after a clean osteotomy, and in patients suffering from transverse mid-shaft fractures of a distal long bone such as the tibia. However in many situations this pattern is not readily identified. In some sites, for example small carpal bones, this is a consequence of the inherent limits of resolution of isotope imaging devices. In others, for example spiral fractures with a butterfly fragment, the limiting factors include the complex anatomy and overlying areas of different activities.

The bone scan has no place in the management of the majority of patients with uncomplicated fractures. It may however be of value when there is clinical or radiological doubt about the presence of a fracture, or its age.

In most sites a repeat x-ray 7–14 days after the initial injury will reveal the majority of fractures not already evident on the initial films. Nevertheless there remains a small percentage of patients in whom uncertainty persists. In these cases a bone scan may be of considerable value (10), as at this time fractures show up as areas of greatly increased uptake clearly distinguishable from soft tissue hyperaemia or adjacent

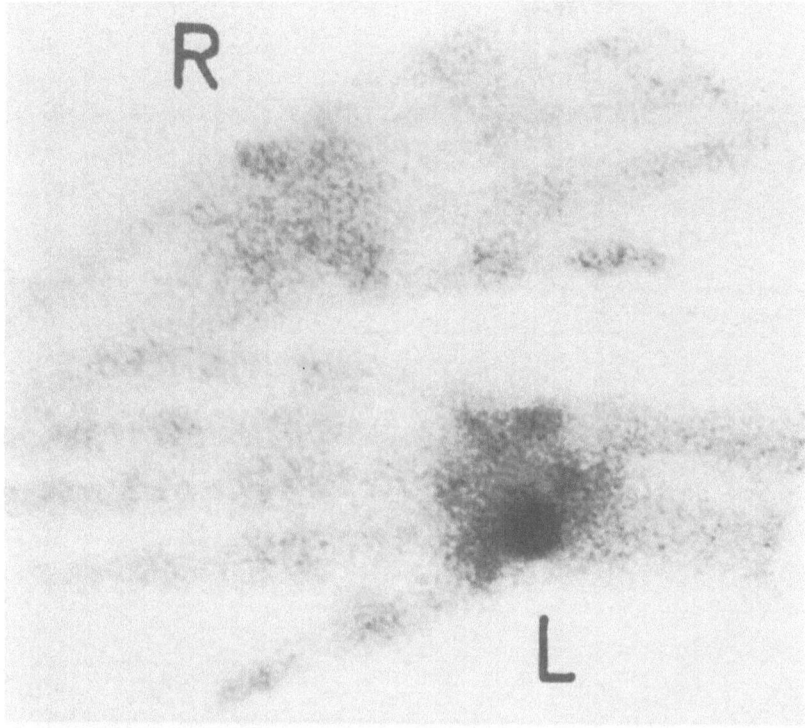

Figure 1a. ^{99m}Tc-MDP bone scan of hands. Patient complained of persistent pain on radial aspect of left wrist for 10 days after fall on outstretched hand. The scan shows increased uptake by the left scaphoid.

bones (Figures 1 and 2). The optimum time to image is probably not less than seven days after injury. Some workers have suggested that imaging may be performed at any time (8) but the possibility of a false negative examination due to soft tissue hyperaemia, or indeed a false positive, cannot be excluded if the examination is performed within the first three days (11).

1.3. *Causes of confusion*

Scans, particularly of small bones such as the carpus, must be interpreted with caution. The scan is an extremely sensitive test for the presence of an abnormality, but is completely non-specific. There are many causes of increased uptake apart from fracture, the most common in the carpus being osteoarthritis, which may be asymptomatic or the

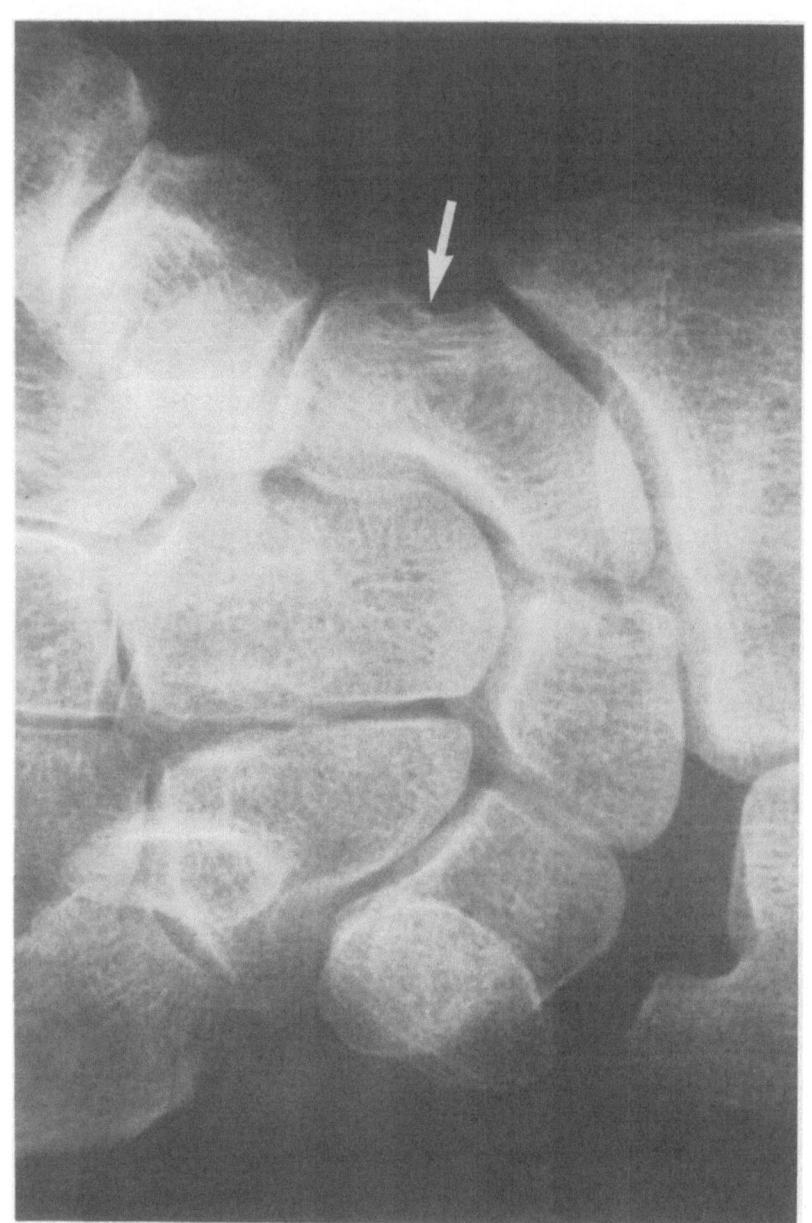

Figure 1b. Radiograph taken on same day as Figure 1a, and initially considered normal. On review an impacted fracture of the distal pole (arrowed) is identified.

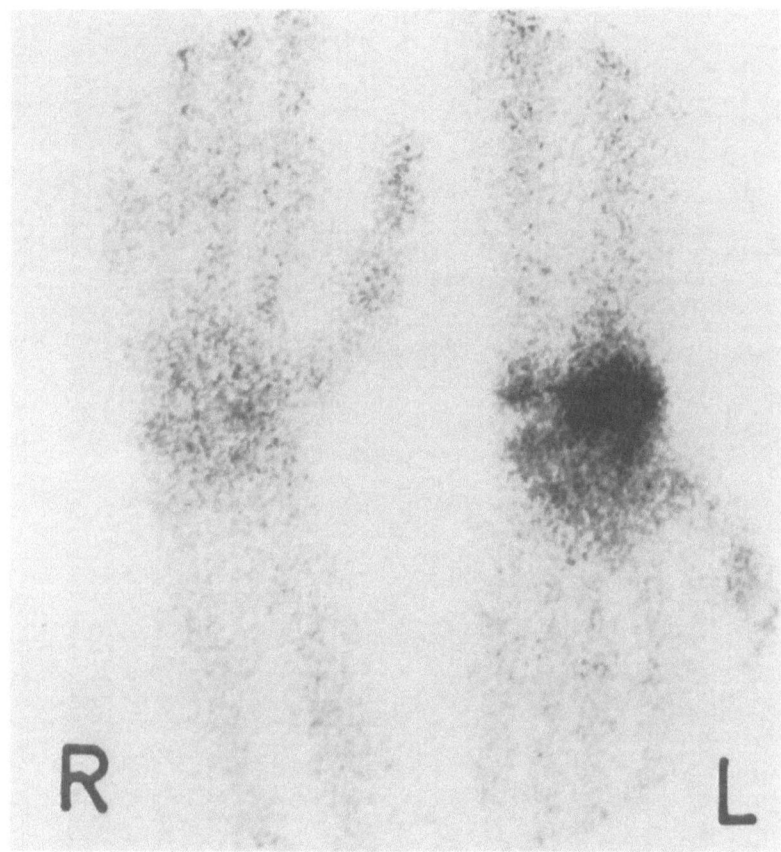

Figure 2. ⁹⁹ᵐTc-MDP bone scan of hands. There was persistent pain despite immobilization for two weeks after fall onto outstretched left hand. In this case the increased uptake is clearly in the distal radius, where the fracture was subsequently confirmed radiologically (styloid process of radius). The slightly increased uptake in the entire carpus is presumably secondary to the reactive hyperaemia around the healing fracture.

cause of only minimal discomfort. This may be visible radiologically. However increased uptake of bone scanning agents normally precedes other (radiological) evidence of "degenerative" arthritis in any joint. Other rare causes of increased uptake include osteochondritis (Figure 3) and melorheostosis.

Paget's disease is usually easier to diagnose, but the existence of x-ray negative Paget's disease has been reported, while scan negative x-ray positive Paget's disease does also exist.

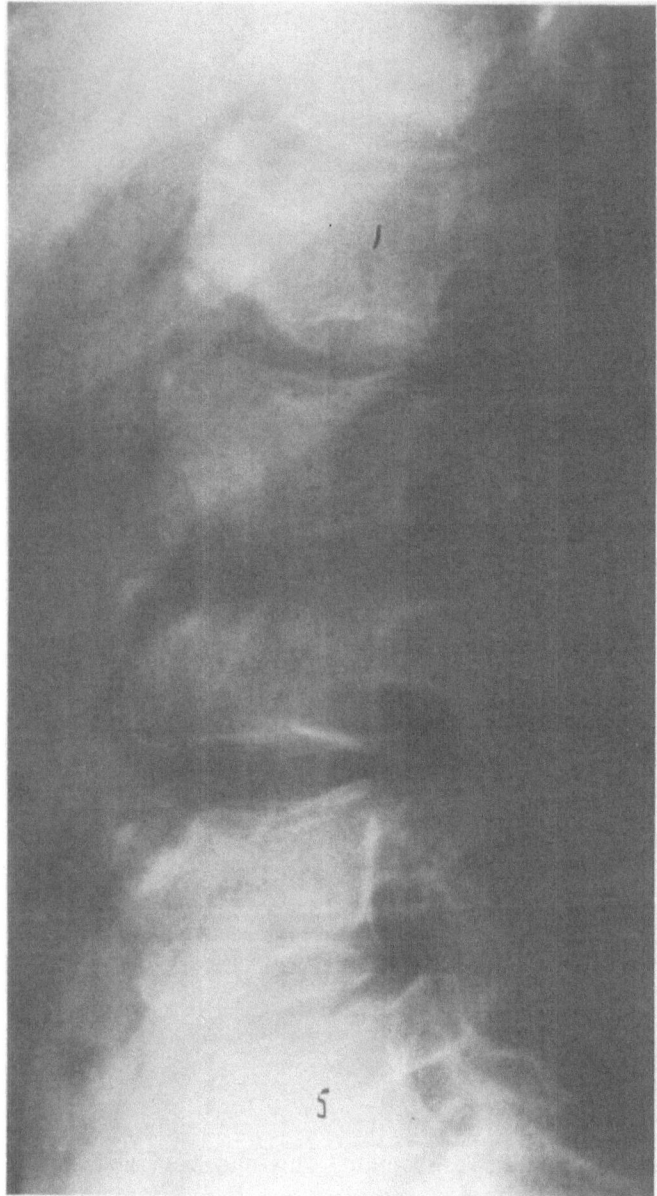

Figure 3a. Lumbar spine of 14-year-old boy with severe persistent lumbar back-ache of many months duration. The film shows the typical end-plate changes of Scheuermann's Disease.

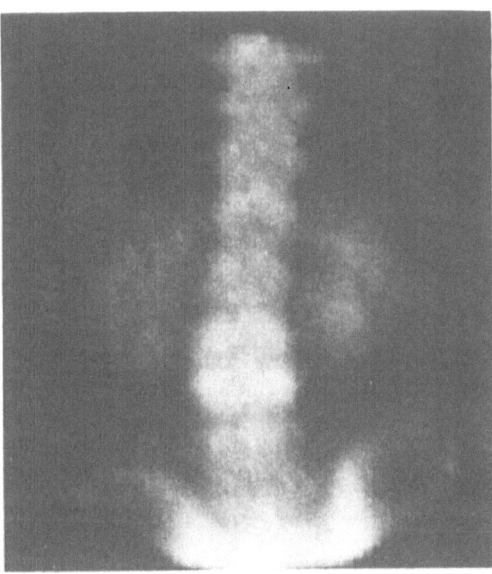

Figure 3b. ^{99m}Tc-MDP bone scan. There is slightly increased uptake in L-3 and L-4, and minimally increased uptake in L-1. The radiographic changes persist for life, but are not associated with persistent symptoms, or a persistently abnormal bone scan. Other pathology was excluded by follow-up of over one year.

It is more difficult to distinguish minor chip fractures and periosteal bruising from a clinically important fracture. It may be sufficient if the bone scan is interpreted in conjunction with the clinical findings, but in many cases it is necessary to resort to high resolution radiography or tomography to make a confident diagnosis (Figures 4 and 5).

1.3.1. *Infection.* Other causes of localised pain and a focal increase of uptake on the bone scan include osteomyelitis. If this is not due to a compound fracture, a whole body scan is mandatory as haematogenous osteomyelitis commonly affects more than one site. In this context it must be remembered that the amount of reaction varies with the organism responsible. The classical pyogenic organisms produce an intense reaction, but some of the less common gram negative organisms may produce relatively little increase of uptake. In these cases a very high quality scan of good statistical content is essential.

1.3.2. *Hyperaemia and osteoporosis.* A further, uncommon, cause of local pain associated with increased uptake of bone scanning agents is

66

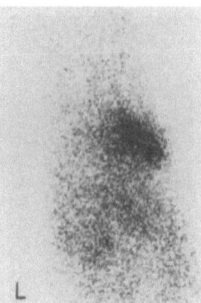

Figure 4a Bone scan of ankle showing increased uptake on the medial aspect. The patient gave a history of persistent pain for four months following a neglected inversion injury.

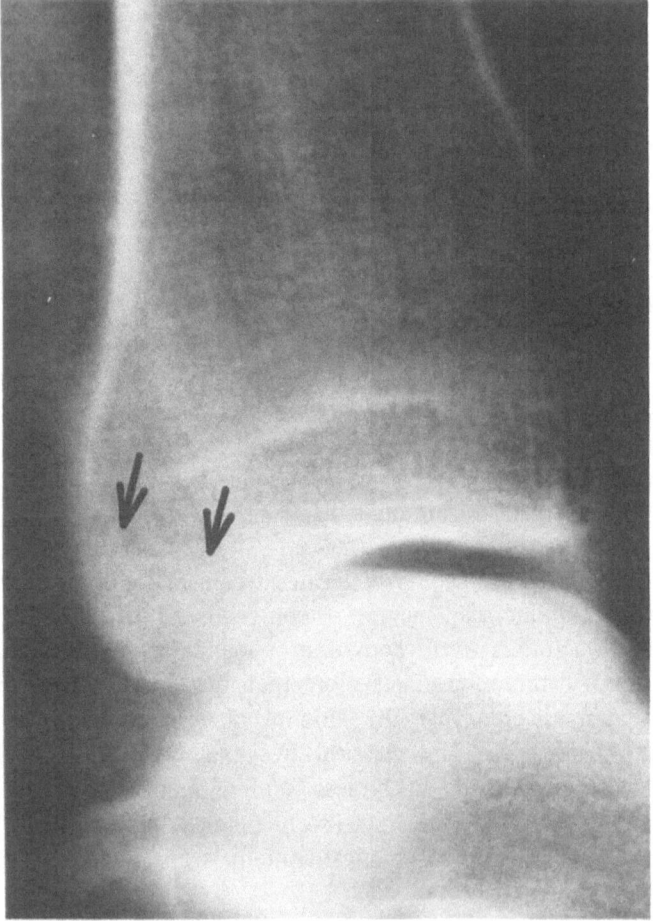

Figure 4b. Plain radiographs were normal. Lateral tomography of the ankle using a fine focus x-ray tube and a hypocycloidal movement revealed this fracture of the posterior malleolus (arrowed), with surprisingly little periosteal reaction.

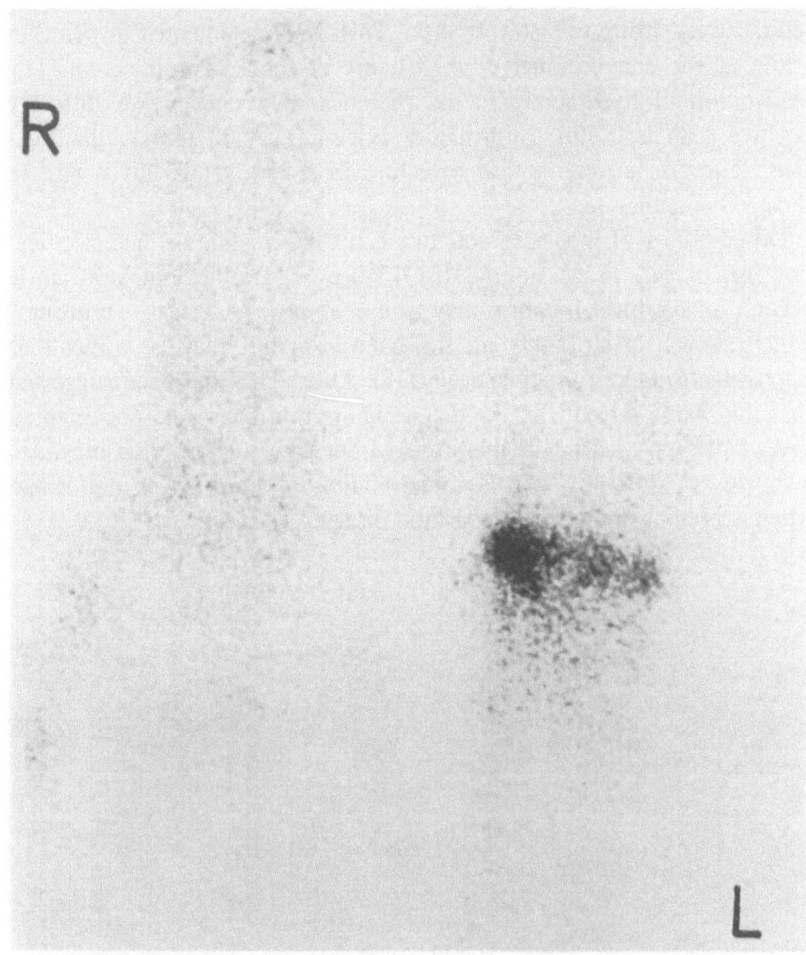

Figure 5. Pain persisting after 7 days immobilization following fall onto outstretched hand. In this case the increased uptake is localized to the trapezoid. Symptoms were relieved by further immobilization in P.O.P., but it was not possible to obtain radiographic confirmation of this uncommon (and clinically not very important) fracture. Compare with Figures 1a and 2.

Sudek's atrophy. Disuse osteoporosis is associated with hyperaemia and therefore locally increased uptake. Sudek's atrophy is an extreme case of this. The diagnosis depends on a combination of clinical, radiographic and radioisotope findings. Hyperaemia may be associated with infection, denervation or soft tissue injury (12, 13). The presence of hyperaemia may be confirmed if imaging is performed immediately after injection of the bone scanning agent before there has been significant clearance of radioactivity from the soft tissues. This is supplemented by further views at the conventional time, 3 hours or more after injection. The recognition of hyperaemia in the presence of a negative or diffusely positive scan is useful confirmatory evidence of soft tissue inflammation. It is also a very noticable feature in osteomyelitis but is rare in most other situations.

Other causes of increased soft tissue uptake include ectopic calcification (14) or soft tissue trauma (15) (Figure 6). Trauma not sufficiently severe to produce fracture may cause minor periosteal "bruising" which shows up strikingly on the bone scan but may be difficult or impossible to identify radiologically (18). Although it has been suggested that this may be useful in the diagnosis of child abuse, no documented cases have appeared in the literature. Minor periosteal reaction may also give rise to difficulty in the interpretation of bone scans performed when searching for occult metastatic disease.

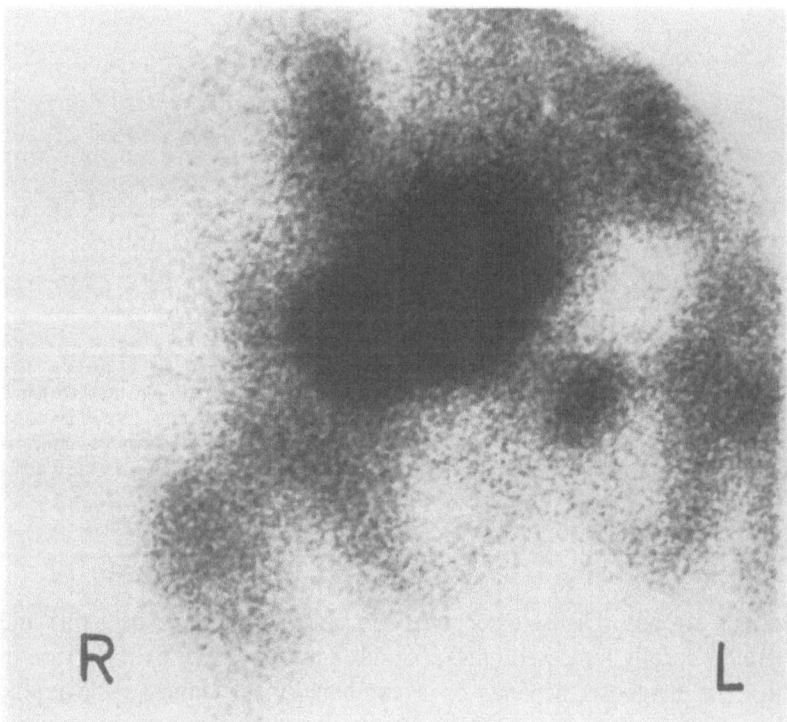

Figure 6a. Bone scan of pelvis of 5-year-old child with pain in the right hip, showing a large area of increased uptake between the triradiate cartilage and the bladder.

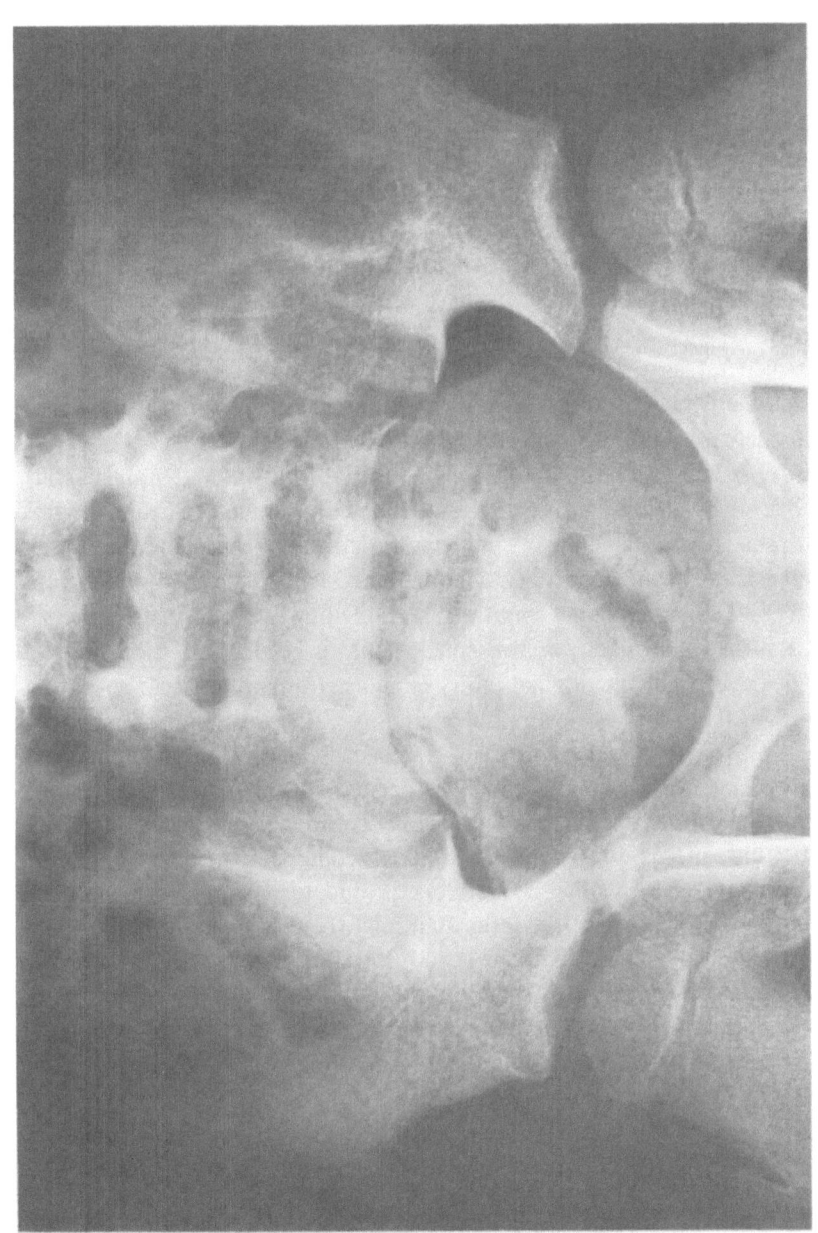

Figure 6b. The radiograph shows a calcified mass in this position. This was confirmed by biopsy to be myositis ossificans. The radiographic appearances have subsequently remained unchanged for two years.

1.4. *The age of a fracture*

The bone scan is of some use in estimating the age of a fracture, but conclusions cannot be drawn too definitely. In one series of 51 patients with crush fractures of the vertebrae, increased uptake of ^{85}Sr was detected in all those examined within six months of fracture, half of those examined between 6 and 18 months later and only one out of 18 examined more than 18 months after injury (16). A similar pattern has been observed in other sites. However increased uptake is detectible with the technetium bone scanning agents for longer after injury than when using ^{85}Sr. It is not clear whether this merely represents the better statistical quality of the scans or a true difference between the two agents.

In general terms the frequency with which increased uptake can be detected on the scan diminishes as the interval between trauma and the scan increases, but in some cases increased uptake persists for many years (17). One extreme case seen by the author showed uptake still visible clearly 37 years after a closed but comminuted fracture of the tibia and fibula. The factors responsible for this persistent increased uptake have never been fully documented. *A priori*, it seems probable that poor alignment and continued remodelling are important factors, but data is inadequate for firm conclusions to be drawn.

The severity of the original injury is another important factor. Abnormally weak bones, for example in patients with osteoporosis or osteomalacia, fracture in response to much less severe trauma than is required for normal bones. This is associated with a shorter duration of uptake detectible on the bone scan (13). The bone scan is therefore of value in patients in whom an isolated collapsed vertebra is found incidentally. If the collapsed vertebra is due to a simple osteoporotic collapse of more than six months standing, there is likely to be little or no increased uptake on the bone scan. More recent collapse is associated with increased uptake. It is therefore not possible to distinguish a recent collapse due to osteoporosis from one due to a metastasis with any useful degree of confidence from the scan alone.

1.5. *Delayed or non-union*

The value of isotope imaging in the detection of delayed union or non-union is a matter of dispute. Some workers have failed to find any difference in uptake between healing fractures and those that subsequently proceed to non-union (19, 20). Other workers have found differences (7, 21, 31).

One recent series studied 100 patients in whom spinal fusion was being performed for scoliosis (22). All the operations were performed by one of two surgeons and following the fusion the patients were immobilised for three months in a plaster jacket. The bone scan was performed on the day that the jacket was removed. All the patients were reexplored the following day to assess union of the grafts. It was found that, although it was easy to distinguish between the technique of the two surgeons, it was impossible to diagnose non-union. However when those patients in whom the scoliosis had increased were rescanned six months later regions of non-fusion were readily detectible. It therefore appears that careful surgery, with meticulous haemostasis, followed by effective immobilisation may be associated with relatively little reactive new bone formation. Only when the region is subjected to stress following the removal of the plaster cast is sufficient focal reaction stimulated to be detectible by the bone scan.

The disagreement of workers at other sites is likely to be due to a complex interaction of multiple factors. Thus when studying patients suffering from simple transverse fractures of the tibia there is little difficulty in seeing the orderly sequence of events described in 1.1. Where more complex fractures are being studied this sequence can rarely be clearly identified.

1.6. *Stress fractures*

Stress fractures are detectible on the bone scan before they are visible radiologically (23). In some patients abnormalities visible on the scan are not subsequently followed by detectible radiological abnormalities (Figure 7). It has been suggested (reasonably but unproven) that microfractures are produced by recurrent stresses and are associated with osteonal remodelling (24). Lamellar bone is reabsorbed and replaced by dense osteonal bone. If the stress is continued at a sufficient level the reabsorption proceeds to a point where bone is weakened and may fracture. However if the bone is rested reabsorption is arrested before this stage is reached. In the latter case there may be correspondingly little or no radiological abnormality. Bone scanning is thus particularly valuable when advising athletes who develop limb pains on training whether or not they should rest, or may safely continue with their exertions (25).

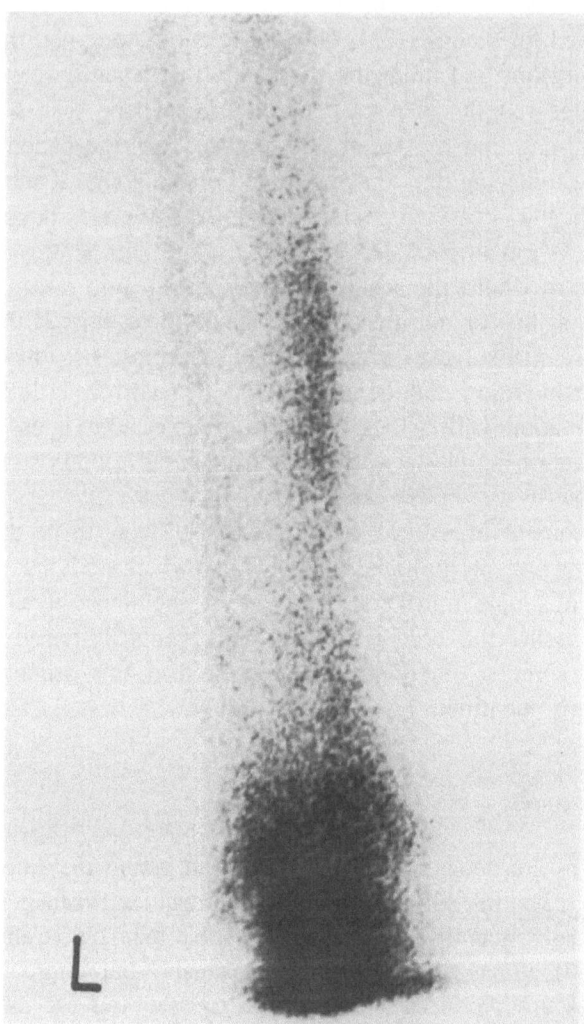

Figure 7a. 18-year old student, physical training instructor, with increasing pain in the left leg. Radiographs were normal. The scan shows a diffuse increase in uptake along the mid-part of the left tibia consistent with stress fracture. The symptoms resolved with rest.

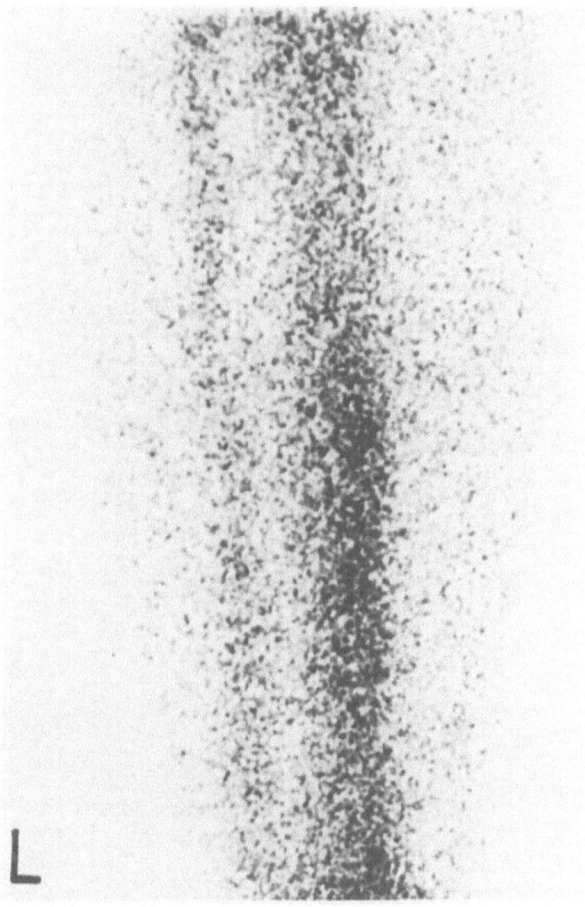

Figure 7b. Four months later the scan is almost normal.

1.7. *Avascular necrosis*

Numerous techniques have been described for assessment of the vascularity of the head of the femur both at operation (by direct injection of tracers) and by scintigraphy (26). The problem is however complicated because avascular necrosis is always associated with revascularisation and repair. No technique is of proven value in the adult. In the adolescent, imaging of the marrow in the femoral head is occasionally of value (27, 28). However there are many causes of local marrow replacement, including old fractures (29), metastatic disease and infarcts (30). Findings must therefore be interpreted with some caution.

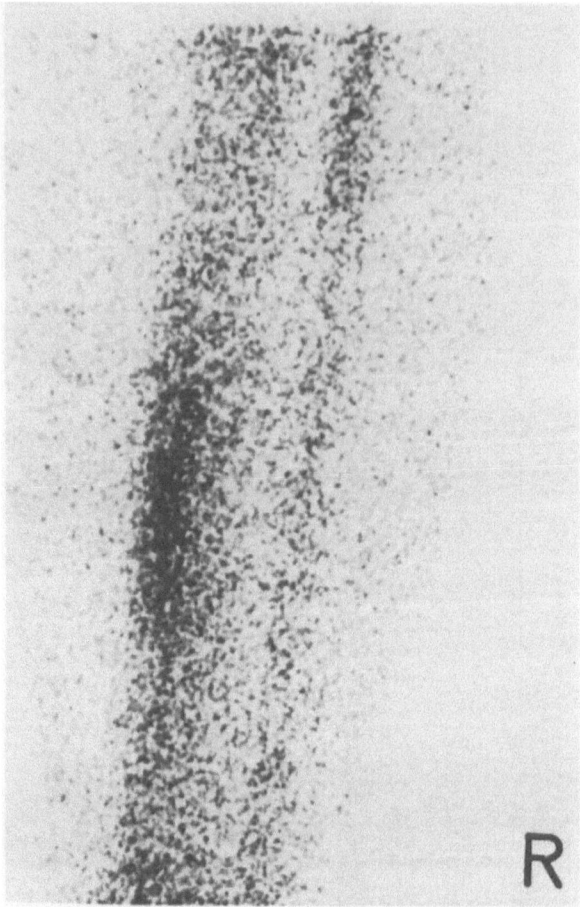

Figure 7c. However, there is now pain in the right leg and the scan shows another incipient stress fracture, this time on the right side.

2. BENIGN BONE TUMOURS

The majority of benign bone tumours can be confidently diagnosed, at least as benign and primary, if due regard is paid to the age and sex of the patient, the site of the lesion and its radiological appearance. A bone scan is rarely if ever indicated, and such experience as there is has largely been accumulated as a result of lesions found incidentally in the course of metastatic surveys. However, as benign bone tumours are most common in children and young adults, whilst metastatic malig-

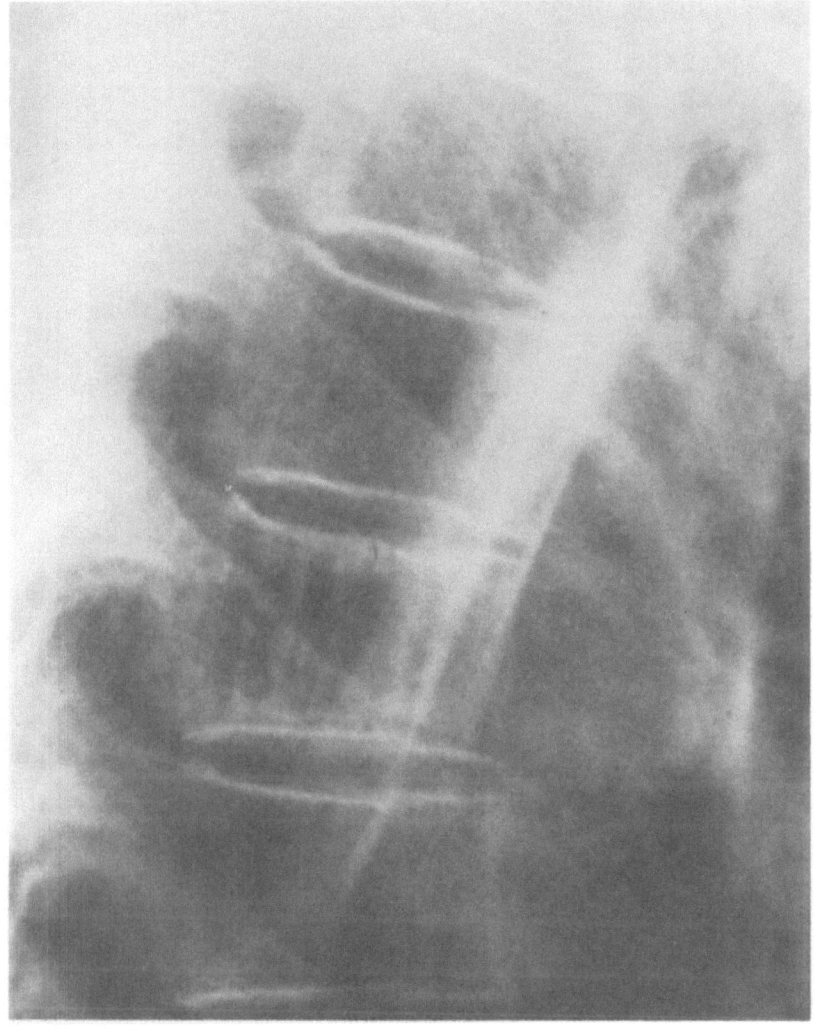

Figure 8a. Haemangioma of T-5, found incidentally during metastatic survey.

nancy is rare in this age group, few workers have seen more than a handful of cases and published reports are sparse, and in general refer to small series.

In general terms it has been suggested that the more vascular a lesion is the more likely it is to be malignant and the greater the uptake of bone scanning agents (32) (Figure 8). Vascularity can be assessed by imaging immediately after injection (33) as for osteomyelitis. This may

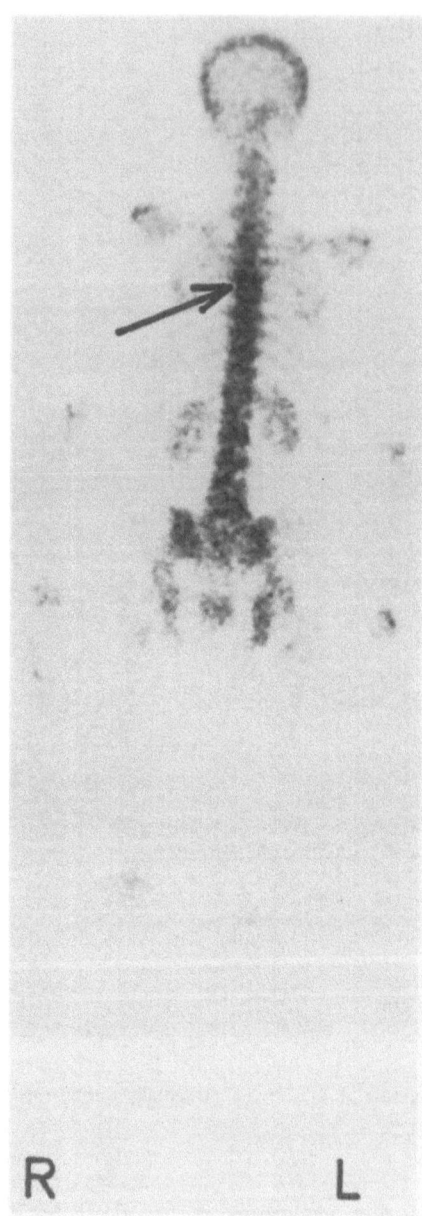

Figure 8b. The bone scan shows only moderately increased uptake (arrowed), despite the vascularity of this benign lesion.

be particularly useful when assessing radiolucent defects. Simple cysts and enchondromata are avascular, and are associated with little or no increase in uptake unless complicated by fracture. Aneurysmal bone cyst is also a "cold" lesion (33) despite its vascularity.

Fibrous dysplasia is most commonly a "hot" lesion (34, 35) although solitary fibrous dysplasia in the humeral head, which is difficult to distinguish on plain film from benign cyst, is "cold". Some lesions of fibrous dysplasia are very vascular. Non-osteogenic fibroma (fibrous cortical defect) produces little or no scintigraphic reaction (33, 36).

Osteochondroma, whether single or multiple, is readily diagnosed clinically and radiologically, although it may be difficilt to detect malignant change at an early stage. During growth uptake of bone-scanning agents parallels that in epiphyseal plates (33). Uptake is however not increased in the majority of lesions in the adult unless there is continued new bone formation or malignant change (37). The bone scan is therefore useful to draw attention to active sites but does not necessarily indicate malignant change. The effect of trauma does not appear to have been studied but is likely to be of considerable importance.

Osteoid osteoma may be difficult to diagnose radiologically, particularly when occurring in the spine, the carpus or the medulla of a long bone. The difficulty may be compounded if there is an atypical clinical history and a low index of suspicion. In the published series (33, 38) and the author's own experience of four cases, there is always markedly increased uptake around the lesion (Figure 9). No false negatives have been recorded even when the nidus was as small as 1 mm^3. There is therefore good reason to perform a bone scan in any patient with localised pain in whom no diagnosis has been made. The scan will not conform the nature of any lesion but will prove that a significant abnormality is present.

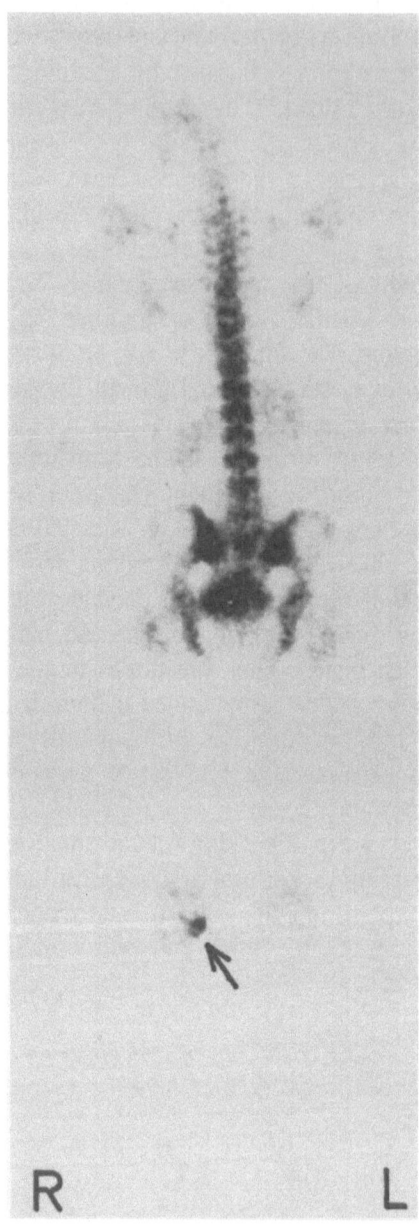

Figure 9a. 32-year-old woman with pain in the right knee for over 6 months. Plain radiographs were considered normal. A whole body scan was performed because of the clinical suspicion that pain was referred from a lesion elsewhere. What it in fact shows is a solitary area of increased uptake on the medial aspect of the right proximal tibia.

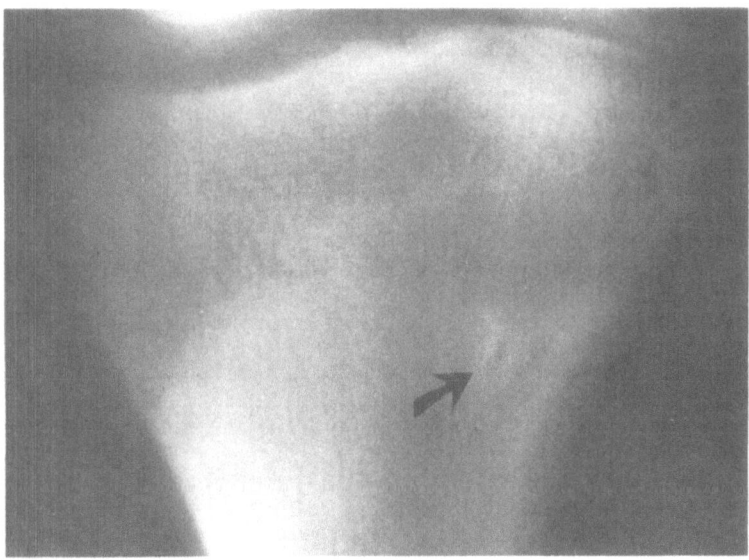

Figure 9b. Hypocycloidal tomography shows a small eccentric nidus with relatively little reaction around it. This is typical of an intramedullary osteoid osteoma, which produces much less sclerosis than the common cortical osteoid osteoma.

REFERENCES

1. Georgi P, Sinn H, Matzku S, Maier-Borst W, Bahk YW: Tierexperimentelle Untersuchungen zur Knockenszintigraphie Nukl Med 9:194-202, 1970.
2. MacDonald NS: Kinetic studies of skeletal metabolism by external counting of radioisotopes: the radioisotope osteogram. J Lab Clin Med 52:541-558, 1958.
3. Bauer GCH, Wendeberg B: External counting of ^{47}Ca and ^{85}Sr in studies of localised skeletal lesions in man. J Bone Jt Surg 41B:558-580, 1959.
4. Heerfordt J, Vistisen L, Bohr H: Comparison of ^{18}F and ^{99m}Tc polyphosphate in orthopaedic bone scintigraphy. J Nucl Med 17:98-103, 1976.
5. Hughes S: The distribution of ^{99m}Tc EHDP in the tissues of the dog and its application in the assessment of fracture healing. Ann R Col Surg Eng 59: 322-327, 1977.
6. Lamel DA: Short term kinetic studies of ^{18}F uptake in normal, x-irradiated and fractured bone. UCLA microfilm order No 71-19, 456, 1971.
7. Gumerman LW, Fogel SR, Goodman MA, Hanley EN, Kappakas GS, Rutkowski R, Levine G: Experimental fracture healing: evaluation using radionuclide bone imaging. J. Nucl Med 19:1320-1323, 1978.
8. Rosenthal L, Hill RO, Chuang S: Observations on the use of ^{99m}Tc phosphate imaging in peripheral bone trauma. Radiology 119:637-641, 1976.
9. Stevenson JS, Bright RW, Dunson GL, Nelson FR: Technetium-99m phosphate bone imaging: a method for assessing bone graft healing. Radiology 110:391-394, 1974.
10. Marty R, Denny JD, McKamey MR, Rowley MJ: Bone trauma and related benign disease: assessment by bone scanning. Sem Nucl Med 6:107-120, 1976.
11. Rolfe EB, Garvie N, Khan MA, Ackery DM: Bone imaging in carpal trauma. Paper read at 7th Annual Meeting of British Nuclear Medicine Soc, 1979.

12. Shim SS, Copp DH, Patterson FP: Bone blood flow in the limb following complete sciatic nerve section. Surg Gynecol Obstet 123:333-335, 1966.
13. Fordham EW, Ramachamdran PC: Radionuclide imaging of osseous trauma. Sem Nucl Med 4:411-429, 1974.
14. Muheim G, Donath A, Rossier AB: Serial scintigrams in the course of ectopic bone formation in paraplegic patients. Am J Roent 118:865-869, 1973.
15. Slutsky LJ, Passalaqua AM, Oster ZH, Braunstein P: Uptake of ^{99m}Tc pyrophosphate in chest wall tissues due to defibrillation. Clin Nucl Med 2:6-7, 1977.
16. Alffram PA, Lindberg L: External counting of ^{85}Sr in vertebral fractures. J Bone Jt Surg 50A:563-569, 1968.
17. Kim HR, Thrall JH, Keys JW: Skeletal scintigraphy following incidental trauma. Radiology 130:447-451, 1979.
18. Iimori M, Hisada K, Suzuki Y: Technetium 99m bone scanning in evaluation of trauma. J Nucl Med 16:538(abs), 1975.
19. Bauer CGH: Radioisotopes and Bone. Editors FC McLean, P Lacroix and AM Budy. Blackwells Oxford, 1962.
20. Johannsen A: Fracture healing controlled by ^{87m}Sr uptake. Acta Orop Scand 44:628-639, 1973.
21. Muheum G: Assessment of fracture healing by serial 87m strontium-scintimetry. Acta Orthop Scand 44:621-627, 1973.
22. MacMaster M, Merrick MV: Use of bone scanning to detect non-union of vertebral fusion in scoliosis. J Bone Jt Surg 62B:65-72, 1980.
23. Wilcox JR, Moniot AL, Green JP: Bone scanning in the evaluation of exercise-related stress injuries. Radiology 123:699-703, 1977.
24. Roub LW, Gumerman LW, Hanley EN, Clark MW, Goodman M, Herbert DL: Bone stress: a radionuclide imaging perspective. Radiology 132:431-438, 1979.
25. Geslien GE, Thrall JH, Espinosa JL, Older RA: Early detection of stress fractures using ^{99m}Tc polyphosphate Radiology 121: 683-687, 1976.
26. Merrick MV: Bone scanning. Brit J Radiol 48:327-351, 1975.
27. Webber MM, Wagner J, Cragin MD: Radionuclide patterns of femoral head disease. Int J Nucl Med Biol 4:167-177, 1977.
28. Turner JH, Martindale AA, Olsthoorn QPM: Technetium 99m antimony colloid bone marrow imaging within 24 hours of subcapital fracture to assess vascularity of the femoral head. J Nucl Med 20:673(abs), 1979.
29. Chafetz N, Slivka J, Taylor A, Alazraki NP, Resnick D, Georgen T: Decreased ^{99m}Tc sulphur colloid activity in healed rib fractures. Radiology 126:735-736, 1978.
30. Kniseley RM: Marrow studies with radiocolloids. Sem Nucl Med 2:71-85, 1972.
31. Alavi A, Desai A, Esterhai J, Brighton C, Dalinka M: Bone scanning in the evaluation of non-united fractures. J Nucl Med 20:647(abs), 1979.
32. Sneppen O, Heerfordt J, Dissing I, Jensen M, Moller J, Norbjerb M: Numerical assessment of bone scintigraphy in primary bone tumours and tumour-like conditions. J Bone Jt Surg 60A:966-969, 1978.
33. Gilday DL, Ash JM: Benign bone tumours. Sem Nucl Med 6:33-46, 1976.
34. Doppelfeld E, Frik W, Fuchs G: Über den Wert der Skeletszintigraphie für die Diagnose der fibrösen Knochendysplasie. Radiologe 18:69-73, 1978.
35. Shuster HL, Sandowsky D, Friedman JM: Radionuclide bone imaging as an aid in the diagnosis of fibrous dysplasia: report of a case. J Oral Surg 37, 267-270, 1979.
36. Brenner RJ, Hattner RS, Lilien DL: Scintigraphic features of nonosteogenic fibroma. Radiology 131:727-730, 1979.
37. Epstein DA, Levin EJ: Bone scintigraphy in hereditory multiple exostoses. Am J Roentgenol 130, 331-333, 1978.
38. Mallens WMC, Pauwels EKJ, Tetteroo QF: Bone scintigraphy as a guide to the diagnosis of osteoid osteoma. Radiologia Clin (Basel) 46:300-306, 1977.

6. SCINTIGRAPHY IN EVALUATING AVASCULAR JOINT DISEASE AND JOINT PROSTHESES

Paul B. Hoffer

Avascular disease
    Legg-Perthes disease
    drug associated avascularity
    post-traumatic disease
Assessment of prosthesis

1. AVASCULAR DISEASE

1.1. *Introduction*

Interruption of blood flow to the femoral head may occur as a result of trauma, medications, underlying small vessel disease or as an idiopathic process of unclear etiology. Tetracycline fluorescence of bone tissue specimens is a well-established method of determining relative bone blood flow but is poorly suited as a noninvasive or preoperative procedure. ^{99m}Tc sulfur colloid has also been used to demonstrate femoral head reticuloendothelial elements and thereby indirectly establish the presence or absence of blood supply, however, this method lacks specificity (1).

It has been documented that ^{18}F and, to a great extent, ^{99m}Tc phosphate compounds localize in bone as a direct function of bone blood flow (2, 3). Since the radiation dose associated with ^{99m}Tc phosphates is modest and excellent images with fine detail can be obtained using the Anger camera and pinhole collimator, this technique has become the method of choice for noninvasive evaluation of vascularity of the femoral head. Specific clinical applications are cited below.

1.2. *Legg-Perthes disease*

Legg-Perthes disease is characterized by loss of vascularity to part or all of the femoral ossification center. It occurs predominantely in male children in the preteen age group. The specific etiology is unknown

Pauwels EKJ, Schütte HE, Taconis WK, eds, Bone scintigraphy, p 81–88.

although genetic predisposition has been observed and precedent minor trauma has been suggested (4). The primary symptoms are pain and limp. The classic initial radiographic findings are shrinking and flattening of the femoral ossification center with expansion of the cartilage joint space. Symptoms frequently preceed radiographic manifestations, however, resulting in diagnostic confusion. Danigelis and associates have observed that all patients with Legg-Perthes disease (with or without radiographic findings) have a characteristic "cold" notch on bone scan involving the superior lateral aspect of the femoral head and best seen on anterior or frog leg views (5, 6). The isotopically cold area, extending medially to a variable degree, was present in all patients with the disease and was seen in no patients with pain due to nonavascular etiology. Ash and co-workers have also been successful in using the presence or absence of femoral head activity to distinguish Legg-Perthes disease from pain due to infection or tumor (7).

Danigelis has also emphasized the value of the bone scan in predicting the radiographic and clinical progress of the disease. Increased radionuclide uptake in the remainder of the ossification center is associated with relatively early reossification of the head and clinical recovery. Absence of increased uptake elsewhere in the ossification center is associated with slower recovery and radiographic reossification. This is true even if increased activity is noted in the epiphysical plate or metaphysical regions.

1.3. *Drug associated avascularity*

Loss of vascularity to the femoral head as a result of small vessel occlusion is a significant complication of steroid therapy and occurs in 10–25% of patients following renal transplantation. The resulting joint changes may require prosthetic replacement of the femoral head. A noninvasive method of evaluating patients following transplantation or during chronic steroid therapy for other diseases may be useful in early detection of vascular compromise and possible prevention of major damage to the head by restriction of weight bearing. Hull and associates have shown that the ^{99m}Tc phosphate bone scan is very sensitive for detection of steroid induced femoral head aseptic necrosis in patients following renal transplantation. Scan changes preceeded radiographic manifestations in about 1/2 of patients while radiographic changes preceeded scan changes in only 1 of 10 patients (8). However, scan changes associated with avascularity may occur transiently in some patients who never develop clinical or radiographic manifestations of loss of vascularity.

1.4. *Post-traumatic disease*

If the blood supply to the femoral head is interrupted due to trauma in an older patient, healing is rare and a total hip arthroplasty is usually the initial procedure of choice. If, however, the blood supply is intact, healing will usually occur and a hip pinning procedure is preferred. Stadalnick and associates have demonstrated that the bone scan is predictive of the femoral head blood supply following trauma (9). Their results correlated well with the presence or absence of tetracycline label in bone biopsy specimens from resected femoral heads. The scan is best performed soon after the injury to avoid confusion with increased activity at the fracture site. Also, the results of the scan must be used cautiously in younger adult patients since revascularization of the avascular femoral head may occur. In this age group serial imaging may be helpful. Illustrative examples are shown in Figures 1 and 2.

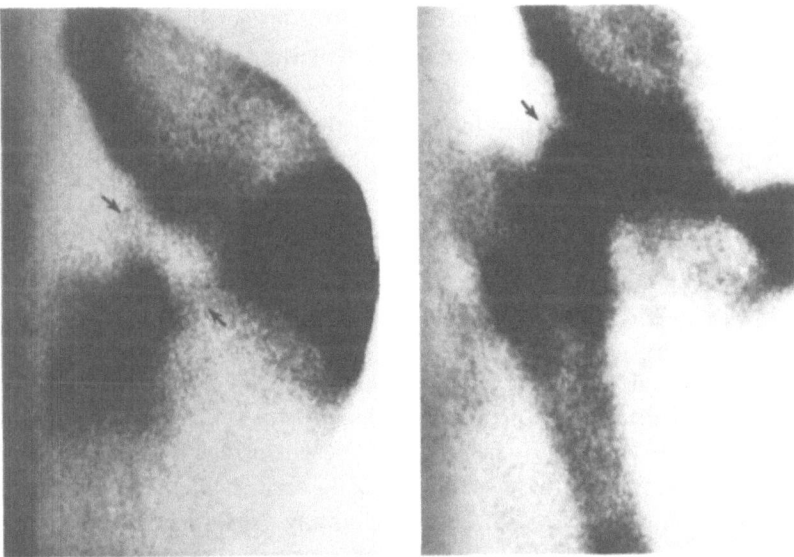

Figure 1   *Figure 2*

Figure 1. ^{99m}Tc MDP bone scan demonstrates absent activity in femoral head (arrows) indicating that the head is avascular. The increased activity in the neck and intertrochanteric regions indicates reactive hyperemia at the fracture site (scanned one week post fracture).

Figure 2. ^{99m}Tc MDP bone scan demonstrates increased activity at fracture site (arrow, neck) and in region of insertion of fixation pins (sub-trochanteric region). Activity in head is slightly increased indicating viability of head (scanned approximately one week post fracture and pinning).

2. ASSESSMENT OF PROSTHESES

2.1. *Introduction*

The total hip arthroplasty is the most common joint prosthesis in current use. Frequently used varieties in the United States are the McKee-Farrer and Charnley-Muller prostheses. It is estimated that in 1977 over 75,000 such prosthesis were implanted. While the most common single indication for use of the prosthesis is degenerative joint disease, other major indications include rheumatoid arthritis, post-traumatic arthritis, avascular necrosis, congenital dislocations and failures of other surgical procedures.

Most complications in the immediate postoperative period are directly related to the surgery or dislocation. These complications are usually easily diagnosed. Following the immediate postoperative period the major complication is prosthetic loosening with or without infection. While this complication occurs in less than 5% of cases, it is important to establish the diagnosis as early as possible since late recognition of loosening and/or infection can result in considerable destruction of femoral stock and compromise future surgical replacement or fusion. Infection and loosening are usually associated with pain. However other minor conditions not requiring surgical intervention may also result in hip pain and it is important to diagnose loosening with or without infection on an objective basis prior to reoperation (10, 11).

2.2. *Diagnosis of loosening prosthesis*

Radiographic detection of prosthetic loosening involves recognition of widening of the lucent zone between cement and bone or demonstration of motion between the bone and prosthesis on cine-fluoroscopy with stress (11). However, these findings usually occur late, after the diagnosis of loosening is well established clinically. Arthrography has been advocated as a diagnostic technique for assessing loosening in patients with hip pain following total hip arthroplasty. Murray and Rodrigo report, however, that this technique is unreliable. They found a 42% incidence of failure of correlation between arthrographic and surgical findings in a group of 12 patients presenting with postoperative hip pain. This included both false positive and false negative studies (2).

In view of the problem in establishing the diagnosis of prosthetic loosening, multiple clinical studies have been conducted to determine the value of radionuclide imaging (13–18). The following general conclusions are common to most or all of these studies.

There is an increase in activity in the femoral and acetabular region adjacent to the prosthesis following implantation which reaches a maximum at approximately 2 months postoperatively and diminishes progressively thereafter. Activity in these regions usually diminishes to normal by six months in assymptomatic patients.

Radionuclide activity is increased in either the femoral and acetabular regions when loosening with or without infection is present and the radionuclide bone scan is thus a highly sensitive test for early detection of loosening. In general, the scan is more sensitive for detection of loosening of the femoral as compared to the acetabular component of the prosthesis.

Blockeel and associates have emphasized that heterotopic bone, which frequently forms in the soft tissues adjacent to the hip joint following surgery, will take up radionuclide on scan (19).

Radionuclide uptake in heterotopic bone may be confused with loosening of the prosthesis. Feith and colleagues note that uptake in heterotopic bone is usually a transient postoperative phenomenon that resolves within 9 months (13). Our experience is that uptake of radionuclide in heterotopic bone is a persistant finding which may be seen many years after surgery (18). It is important to note that the study performed by Feith used [87m]Sr while we used ^{99m}Tc MDP. Another major cause of confusion is radionuclide uptake in the calcar region which is a nonspecific finding (16).

In our experience, the most reliable method of diagnosis of loosening of the femoral component of a total hip prosthesis is by evaluation of radionuclide uptake in the femoral bone adjacent to the *distal* tip of the prosthesis. Increased activity in this region was observed in 15 of 16 cases of femoral component loosening and only 3 of 16 controls (18) (see Figures 3 and 4).

In spite of the imperfections of the bone scan in diagnosing prosthetic loosening it is probably the most reliable method of early confirmation of the diagnosis in patients with hip pain following total hip arthroplasty.

There is still no clinically proven reliable method to distinguish loosening due to infection from sterile loosening. While Williamson has suggested that a diffuse pattern of uptake about the prosthesis is frequently seen in association with infection, this finding awaits further clinical confirmation (20).

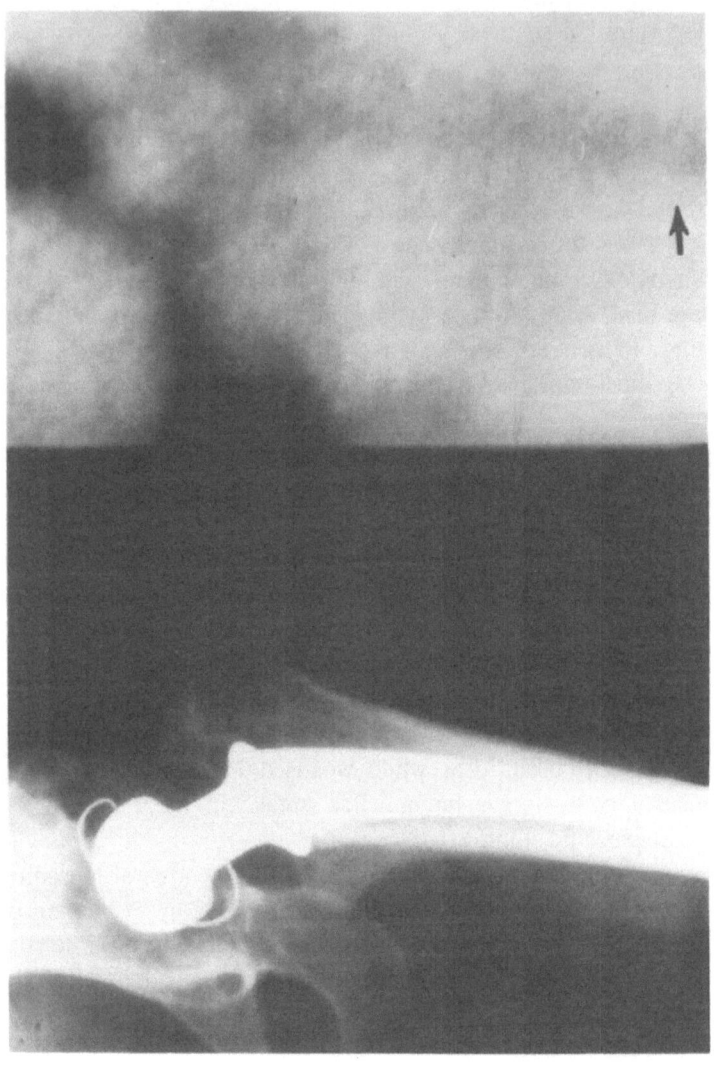

Figure 3. **Radiograph and** ^{99m}**Tc MDP bone scan of patient 6+ months post insertion of prosthesis. Absence of** activity in region of distal femoral prosthetic component (arrow) strongly suggests the prosthesis is not loose. Persistent pain resulted in surgery which demonstrated an intact prosthesis.

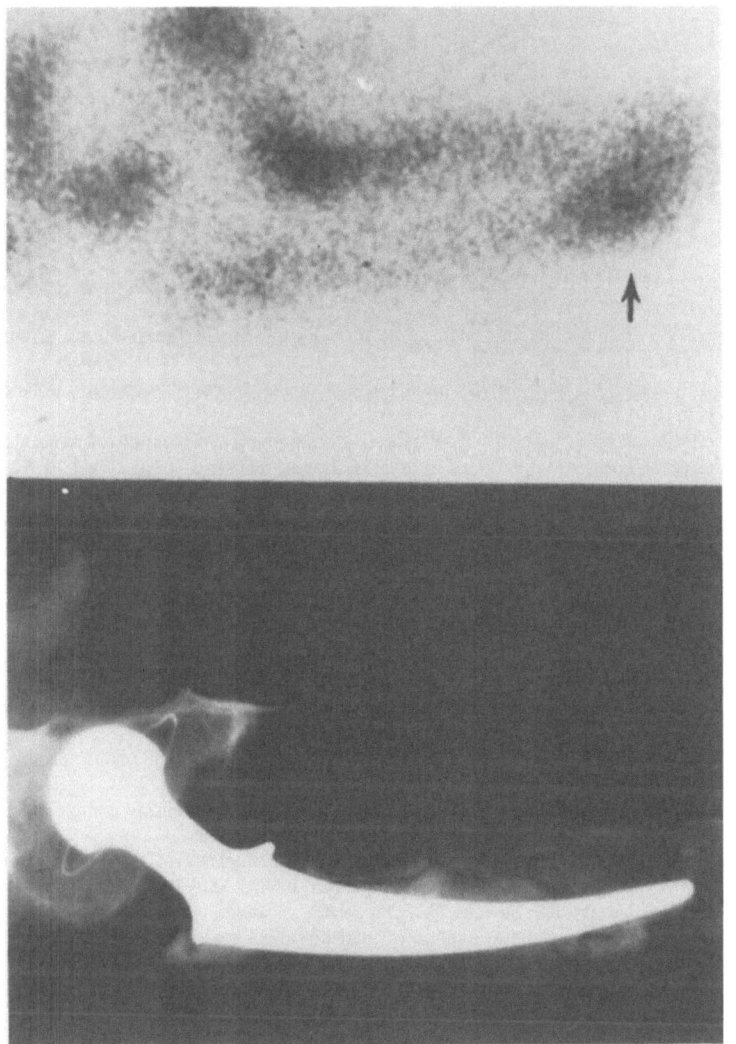

Figure 4. Radiograph and ^{99m}Tc MDP bone scan of patient 6+ months post insertion of prosthesis. Activity in region of distal portion of femoral component (arrow) suggests loosening (surgically proven).

REFERENCES

1. Webber NM, Wagner J, Cragin MD: Radionuclide patterns of femoral head disease. Int J Nucl Biol Med 4:167-177, 1977.
2. Van Dijke D, Anger HO, Yano Y, Bozzini C: Bone Blood flow shown with ^{18}F and the positron camera. Am J Physiol 209: 65-70, 1965.
3. Genant HK, Bautovich GJ, Singh M, Lathrop KA, Harper PV: Bone-seeking radionuclides: an in vivo study of factors affecting skeletal uptake. Radiology 113:373, 1974.
4. Caffey J: Pediatric x-ray diagnosis, 5th edition year book, Medical Publishers Inc, Chicago, 1967, p 904.
5. Danigelis JA, Fisher RL, Ozonoff MB, Sziklas JJ: ^{99m}Tc-polyphosphate bone imaging in Legg-Perthes disease. Radiology 115:407-413, 1975.
6. Danigelis JA: Pinhole imaging in Legg-Perthes disease: further observations. Semin Nucl Med 6:69-82, 1976.
7. Ash Jm, Gilday DL, Reilly BJ: Pinhold imaging of hip disorders in children. J Nucl Med 16:512-513, 1975.
8. Hull A, Hattner RS, Vincente F: Prospective scintigraphic evaluation of avascular necrosis (AVN) of the femoral head in renal transplant recipients. J Nucl Med 20:646, 1979.
9. Stadalnick RC, Riggins RL, D'Ambrosia R, DeNardo GL: Vascularity of the femoral head: ^{18}Fluorine scintigraphy validated with tetracycline labeling. Radiology 114:663-666, 1975.
10. Murray WR: Results in patients with total hip replacement arthroplasty. Clin Orthopedics & Related Research 95:80-90, 1973.
11. Dolinskas C, Campbell RE, Rothman R: The painful Charnley total hip replacement. Am J Roentgenol 121:61-68, 1974.
12. Murray WR, Rodrigo JJ: Arthrography for the assessment of pain after total hip replacement. J Bone Joint Surg 57A:1060-1065, 1975.
13. Feith R, Slooff TJJF, Kazem I, Van Rens Th JG: Strontium ^{87m}(SR) bone scanning for the evaluation of total hip replacement. J Bone Joint Surg 58:79-83, 1976.
14. Campeau RJ, Hall MF, Maile A Jr: Detection of total hip arthroplasty complications with Tc-99m pyrophosphate. J Nucl Med 17:526, 1976 (Ab).
15. Creutzig H: Bone imaging after total replacement arthroplasty of the hip joint: a follow-up with different radiopharmaceuticals. Eur J Nucl Med 1:177-180, 1976.
16. Gelman MI, Coleman RE, Stevens PM, Davey BW: Radiography, radionuclide imaging, and arthrography in the evaluation of total hip and knee replacement. Radiology 128:677-682, 1978.
17. McInerny DP, Hyde ID: Technetium ^{99m}TC pyrophosphate scanning in the assessment of the painful hip prosthesis. Clin Radiol 29:513-517, 1978.
18. Weiss PE, Mall JC, Hoffer PB, Murray WR, Rodrigo JJ, Genant HK: Technetium-99m Methylene Diphosphonate imaging in the evaluation of total hip prosthesis. Radiology, 133: 727-729, 1979.
19. Blockeel R, Hollaert P, Schelstraete K: The sleeve phenomenon in bone scintigraphy: an early demonstration of paraarticular ossification after total hip replacement. J Belge De Radiologie 5:423-426, 1975.
20. Williamson BRJ, McLaughlin RE, Gwo-Jaw W, Miller CW, Teates CD, Bray ST: Radionuclide bone imaging as a means of differentiating loosening and infection in patients with a painful total hip prosthesis. Radiology 133:723-725, 1979.

PART III

BONE SCINTIGRAPHY
IN METABOLIC DISORDERS

7. BONE DENSITOMETRY IN LONG-TERM DIALYSIS PATIENTS

CHRIS ALBERTS

The introduction of long-term regular haemodialysis by Scribner(1) in 1960 made it possible for renal failure patients to survive longer than was possible when conservative measures alone were employed. However, with the artificial kidney therapy skeletal disorders still can influence the quality of life and contribute to the morbidity of these patients. Various haemodialysis centres report a differing incidence, nature and severity of skeletal disease, resulting from a combination of disturbed calcium, phosphorus and vitamin D metabolism and different dialysate calcium concentrations. Evolution of the bone disease during regular haemodialysis depends on the state of the skeleton when the patients begin haemodialysis. Early treatment aimed at correcting hypocalcaemia, vitamin D deficiency and concurrent hyperphosphataemia may ensure that patients on haemodialysis remain free of musculoskeletal symptoms. The diagnosis of haemodialysis bone disease should be made by the combination of clinical, biochemical, radiological and histopathological findings. Defective mineralization with the reduction of bone mass is the most characteristic feature of haemodialysis bone disease. The histological manifestations are secondary hyperparathyroidism with osteitis fibrosa, hyperosteoidosis with osteomalacia, osteoporosis, or combinations of these multiple abnormalities. Clinical symptoms, such as irritated red eyes, pruritus, muscular weakness, diffuse and local skeletal pain and spontaneous fractures, are signs of advanced haemodialysis bone disease (2–4).

The best method for studying skeletal disorders is bone histology, but a variety of techniques have been developed which can estimate the amount of mineral in the skeleton. Radiographic measurements (especially the determination of the " metacarpal index ") and direct photon absorptiometry are the only techniques suitable for the routine analysis of quantitative bone changes. Unlike bone histology, these techniques are unsuitable for diagnostic purposes. Their value lies in the serial assessment of skeletal status. They may yield information about bone loss and provide indirect assessments of the value of therapeutic manipulations, such as varying the dialysate calcium concentration, treat-

Pauwels EKJ, Schütte HE, Taconis WK, eds, Bone scintigraphy, p 91–97.

ment with vitamin D and calcium, and parathyroid surgery. A source of concern when regional assessment of bone loss is made in haemodialysis patients, is that changes in one part of the skeleton may not reflect changes occurring elsewhere. In order to examine this possibility and the value of regional techniques, such as direct photon absorptiometry, we have measured forearm bone mineral content and bone density in long-term haemodialysis patients and compared this to clinical symptoms, biochemistry and histology of iliac crest bone biopsies.

1. TECHNIQUES

In this study we have used the Cameron-Sorenson (5) technique of scanning the distal third of the radius with a well-collimated photon beam from a monochromatic 1-125 source (Norland-Cameron Bone Mineral Analyzer). The forearm is placed in a limb holder between two flat parallel surfaces. The tissue cover is made uniform by a water-filled bag around the forearm. The detector and 1-125 source are driven across the forearm by a motor drive system and a computer module calculates the bone mineral content and width of the radius. The *bone width* (W) is determined by the rapid attenuation of photons at both bone edges and the *bone mineral content* (BMC) is proportional to the area under the absorption curve. Dividing BMC by W partially corrects for skeletal size and provides an expression equivalent to bone density in g per sq cm. This technique for determining bone mineral content and bone density in vivo has proved to be a reproducible and accurate method for frequent analysis of changes in bone mass (6-7).

The *bone mineral content* (BMC) and *bone density* (BMC/W) were measured in 38 patients known to the St. Lucas Hospital in Amsterdam as suffering from chronic renal failure treated by regular haemodialysis. All patients had been established on regular haemodialysis for 2 to 7 years. They had been kept on a normal protein diet and were being treated with aluminium hydroxide, vitamin D and calcium supplements. Haemodialysis was performed with disposable Cordis Dow Hollow Fiber dialyzers, two to three times a week; the calcium concentration of the dialysate was 7.0 mg/100 ml. All patients had periodic physical examinations, iliac crest biopsies every six months and serum calcium, phosphorus and alkaline phosphatase evaluations at 6-weekly intervals. A number of haemodialysis patients, in whom the dialyzer and the duration and frequency of treatment were kept constant, had multiple bone mineral content (BMC) and bone density (BMC/W) measurements during $2\frac{1}{2}$ years of study.

2. RESULTS

The results of the bone mineral content (BMC) and bone density (BMC/W) measurements in the chronic haemodialysis patients were compared to the values in a sex- and age-matched group of 46 normal subjects (21 men and 25 women) who had no evidence of bone disease (8).

The bone mineral content (BMC) varied widely, from 0.58 to 1.15 g/cm in the female dialysed group and 0.63 to 1.43 g/cm in the male dialysed group. The variation of bone mineral content is due in part to the degree of mineral loss but also reflects sex, age and size of the haemodialysis patient. Therefore, we have used the bone density (BMC/W) value, which includes the correction for skeletal size. The majority of haemodialysis patients showed a decreased bone density (BMC/W), compared to values found in normal adults of corresponding sex and age group (Figure 1). These results confirm other investigations (9–11). In the group of 19 female patients with ages ranging from 17 to 65 years, the mean bone density was 0.63 ± 0.09 g per sq cm (range 0.45–0.77 g per sq cm). The 19 male haemodialysis patients, aged from 18 to 64 years, had bone density measurements of 0.54–0.84 g per sq cm, mean 0.70 ± 0.08 g per sq cm. The mean values for both groups of patients were significantly ($p < 0.001$) lower than those of the control groups of normal subjects (Table 1).

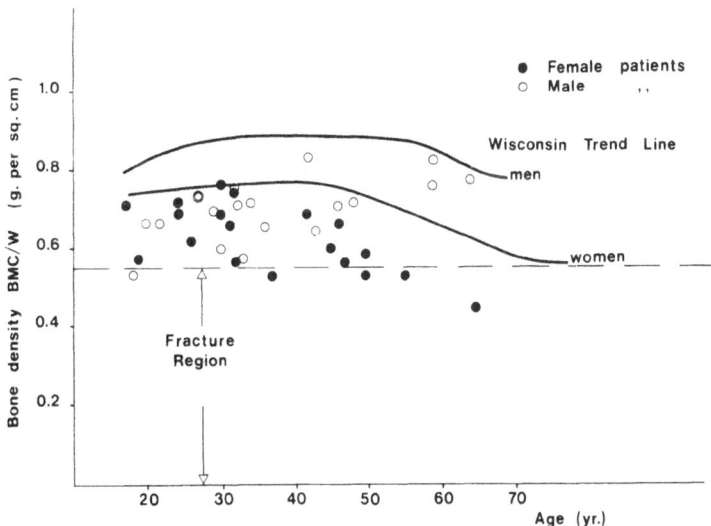

Figure 1. Bone density (BMC/W) in 19 female and 19 male haemodialysis patients compared to the Wisconsin normal trend lines (8).

94

Table 1. Bone mineral content (BMC) and bone density (BMC/W) in long-term haemo-dialysis patients and normal subjects (8).

			Age (yr)	BMC (g/cm)	BMC/W (g/cm²)
Dialysis patients					
	19 women		17–65	0.58–1.15	0.45–0.77
		mean	37	0.81	0.63
38					
	19 men		18–64	0.63–1.43	0.54–0.84
		mean	37	1.08	0.70
Normal subjects					
	25 women		16–56	0.69–1.14	0.62–0.80
		mean	32	0.94	0.73
46					
	21 men		18–62	0.95–1.63	0.70–1.01
		mean	40	1.30	0.84

3. DISCUSSION

The bone density measurements in the control group of 46 normal subjects were comparable to the results of the Wisconsin population studies (12). It should be mentioned that women lose more bone than men after forty-five years of age. Therefore, the male trend line decreases less rapidly than the female trend line with increasing age.

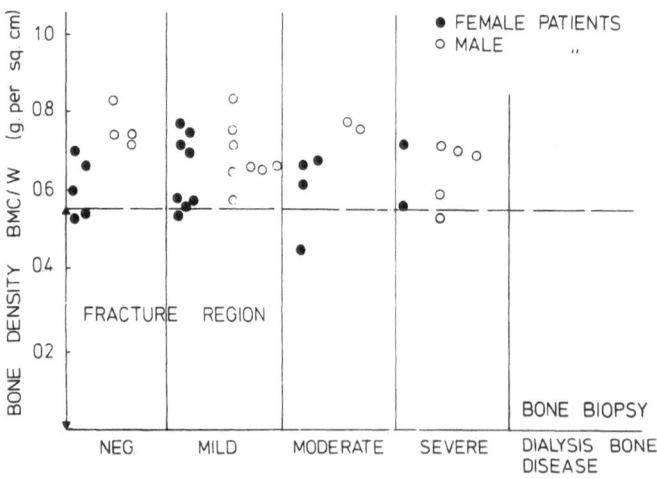

Figure 2. Bone density (BMC/W) values in long-term haemodialysis patients, 38, compared to the iliac crest bone biopsy findings.

In this series of long-term haemodialysis patients, there were 5 patients with bone density values below 0.55 g per sq cm, a value with high probability for bone fractures as obtained by Smith (13) in a 3-year study of normal and osteoporotic women.

The follow-up of the patients on long-term haemodialysis treatment have shown that the regional assessment of bone density by photon absorptiometry did not always correlate with the severity of haemodialysis bone disease, including clinical symptoms, change in biochemistry and/or histopathology of bone biopsies (Figure 2). The results of bone density measurements were misleading in some patients on regular haemodialysis. Eight patients had symptomatic haemodialysis bone disease. However, the majority, 5, of these patients showed no extreme decrease in bone density values (Table 2). Intensive treatment with vitamin D and oral calcium supplements was followed by either reversal of clinical symptoms and improvement of bone biopsy findings and/or correction of serum calcium, phosphorus and alkaline phosphatase. In contrast to the clinical improvement the osteopenia, determined by bone density measurements with 1–125 photon absorptiometry, remained at the same level. The results suggest that the forearm assessment of bone loss do not accurately reflect changes occurring elsewhere in the skeleton of the chronic haemodialysis patient.

The clinical follow-up of regular haemodialysis patients, 17, during $2\frac{1}{2}$ year demonstrated that the response of haemodialysis bone disease to treatment with vitamin D and calcium is not uniform, and that in this

Table 2. Bone density (BMC/W) and iliac crest biopsy in 8 long-term haemodialysis patients with clinical signs and symptoms of haemodialysis bone disease (8).

Patient	Age	BMC/W (g/cm^2)	Bone biopsy osteodystrophy	Clinical signs and symptoms
Male patients				
1 [b]	43	0.65	+	multiple rib fractures; pain in foot and ankles
2	33	0.58	+	pain in right hip
3	59	0.77	+	rib pain
4	36	0.66	+	rib pain
5	30	0.60	+ +	scapula fracture
6 [a]	20	0.67	+	pain in ankles
Female patients				
7	42	0.69	+	pain in foot
8	45	0.60	+	spontaneous march fracture

[a] Parathyroidectomy, 1969.
[b] Parathyroidectomy, 1974.

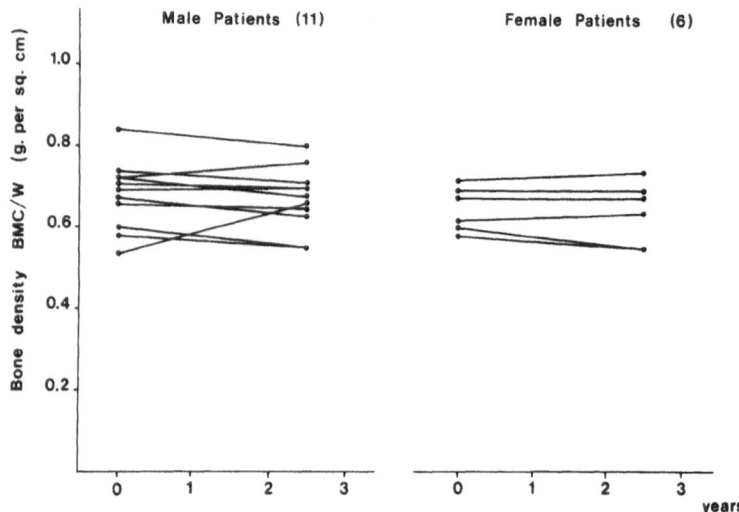

Figure 3. Bone density (BMC/W) values in long-term haemodialysis patients during and after $2\frac{1}{2}$ year haemodialysis treatment (8)

series some regression of haemodialysis bone disease may have taken place. Despite a sustained return to normal calcium and phosphorus metabolism, decreased mineralization of the appendicular skeleton can persist (Figure 3). Whether this finding is an indicator of an irreversible component of haemodialysis bone disease cannot be stated. Also, it is uncertain whether the results of this study may have been influenced by the fact of long-term haemodialysis treatment.

Bone density measurements by photon absorptiometry may nevertheless be useful in the follow-up of patients with chronic renal failure from the beginning of haemodialysis and after kidney transplantation. However, the bone density values have to be considered together with other clinical data in reaching a final interpretation of bone disease associated with haemodialysis.

ACKNOWLEDGEMENTS

My thanks are due to the staff of the Dialysis Unit for assistance, to Mrs. E. Busemann Sokole for review of this paper, to Mr. C. Bor for reproducing the figures and to Miss E.C. Drost for typing the manuscript.

The Norland-Cameron Bone Mineral Analyzer was kindly supplied by the Optische Industrie "De Oude Delft", Delft, The Netherlands. Figures 1 and 3, Table 2 and parts of the text have been reproduced with permission from the European Journal of Nuclear Medicine 4: 27–31, 1979.

REFERENCES

1. Scribner BH, Buri R, Caner JEA, Hegström R, Burnell JM: The treatment of chronic uremia by means of intermittent haemodialysis: a preliminary report. Trans Amer Soc Artific Intern Org 6:114, 1960.
2. Kennedy AC: Maintenance dialysis. In: Renal disease; Black D, Jones NF (eds), Oxford, Blackwell Scientific Publications, 1979 (4th ed), p 523-548.
3. Deluca HF, Avioli LV: Renal osteodystrophy. In: Renal disease; Black D, Jones NF (eds), Oxford, Blackwell Scientific Publications, 1979 (4th ed.), p 766-803.
4. Stanbury SW: Azotaemic renal osteodystrophy. In: Clinics in endocrinology and metabolism: calcium metabolism and bone disease; MacIntyre I (ed), London, Saunders Company Ltd, 1972, p 267-304.
5. Cameron JR, Sorenson J: Measurement of bone mineral. In vivo: an improved method. Science 142:230-232, 1963.
6. Mazess RB, Cameron JR, O'Connor R, Knutzen D: Accuracy of bone mineral measurement. Science 145:388-389, 1964.
7. Cameron JR, Mazess RB, Sorenson JA: Precision and accuracy of bone mineral determination by direct photon absorptiometry. Invest Radiol 3:141-150, 1968.
8. Alberts C: I-125 photon absorptiometric analysis of bone density in patients on regular dialysis treatment. Eur J Nucl Med 4:27-31, 1979.
9. Atkinson PJ, Hancock DA, Acharya VN, Parsons FM, Procter EA, Reed GW: Changes in skeletal mineral in patients on prolonged maintenance dialysis. Br Med J 4:519-522, 1973.
10. Griffiths HJ, Zimmerman RE, Bailey G, Snider R: The use of photon absorptiometry in the diagnosis of renal osteodystrophy. Diagn Radiol 109:277-281, 1973.
11. Mayor GH, Sanchez TV, Garn SM: Determining bone mineral status in renal patients – the use of photon absorptiometry. Dialysis – Transplantation 5:36-39, 1976.
12. Mazess RB, Cameron JR: Bone mineral content in normal U.S. whites. International conference on bone mineral measurement, Chicago, Illinois, October 12-13, 1973.
13. Smith EL: Bone changes with age and physical activity. Thesis, University of Wisconsin, 1971.

8. BONE SCANNING AND 24-HOUR WHOLE BODY RETENTION OF DIPHOSPHONATE IN THE EVALUATION OF METABOLIC BONE DISEASE

Ignac Fogelman and Rodney G Bessent

Bone scan appearances
    osteoporosis
    osteomalacia
    renal osteodystrophy
    primary hyperparathyroidism
Bone scanning compared with radiology
Semi-quantitative evaluation of the bone scan image
Quantitation of skeletal uptake of radiopharmaceutical

Radiology of the skeleton reveals the net result of bone resorption and formation and before a lesion becomes visible it has to be approximately 1.5 cms in size with loss of around 50% of the local mineral content (1). The bone scan on the other hand depends upon osteoblastic activity and to a lesser extent vascularity for uptake of tracer onto bone (2). When the skeleton is invaded by tumour there is a local increase in osteoblastic activity with increased blood flow and the bone scan may appear positive 6 months, 1 year or on occasion 18 months before changes are recognised on x-ray. The bone scan in now well established in the evaluation of patients with metastatic disease where its superiority over radiology is well recognised (3, 4).

1. BONE SCAN APPEARANCES IN THE METABOLIC BONE DISORDERS

As skeletal uptake of tracer is related to osteoblastic activity and blood flow, the bone scan essentially displays a functional image of skeletal metabolic activity and one would predict that the bone scan would be of considerable value in metabolic bone disease. However, in the metabolic bone disorders the skeleton is usually diffusely involved by the metabolic process and characteristically focal abnormalities are not seen. A recognition of abnormality then depends upon a subjective impression of increased tracer uptake throughout the whole skeleton and this may not always be apparent. As more experience is gained with bone scanning, patterns of bone scan abnormality and certain metabolic features

Pauwels EKJ, Schütte HE, Taconis WK, eds, Bone scintigraphy, p 99–109.
Copyright © 1981 Martinus Nijhoff Publishers bv, The Hague/Boston/London. All rights reserved.

are becoming recognised in the metabolic bone disorders (5–8). We have described 7 such metabolic features on the bone scan that we believe to be characteristic of the metabolic bone diseases in general (9) (Table 1) (Figures 1–6).

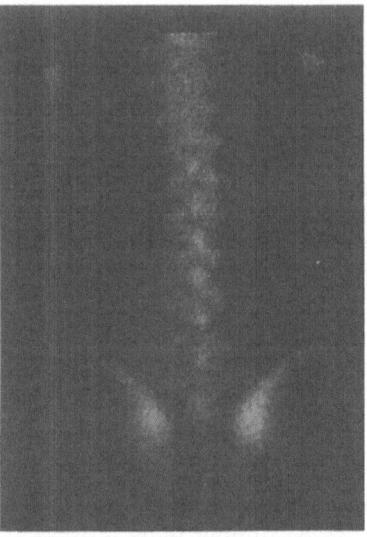

Figure 1. Bone scan view of posterior spine demonstrating high tracer uptake in axial skeleton and absent kidney images.

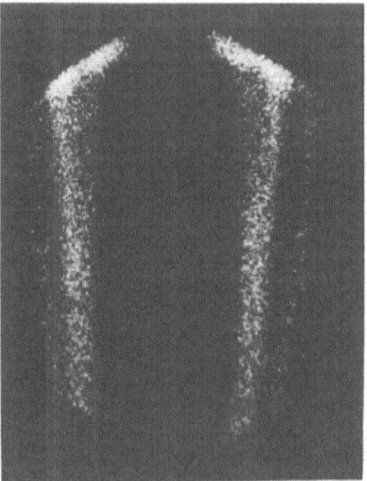

Figure 2. Increased tracer uptake is seen in lower limbs. Note fibulae are clearly visualised.

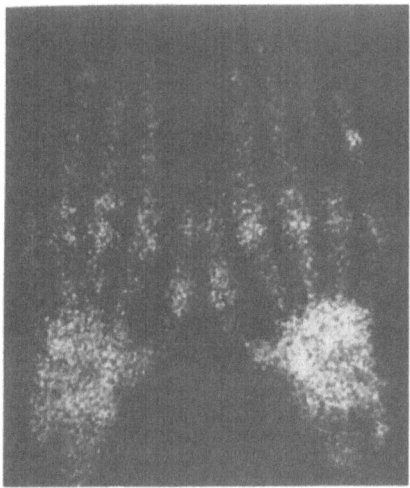

Figure 3. Scan of wrists and hands showing increased peri-articular uptake of tracer.

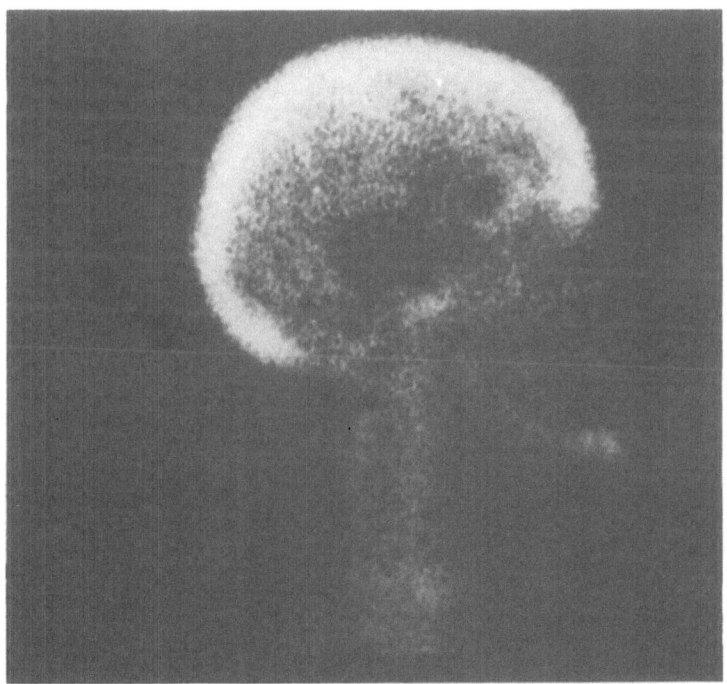

Figure 4. Lateral view of skull and facial bones demonstrating increased tracer uptake by calvarium. The mandible is clearly visualised.

102

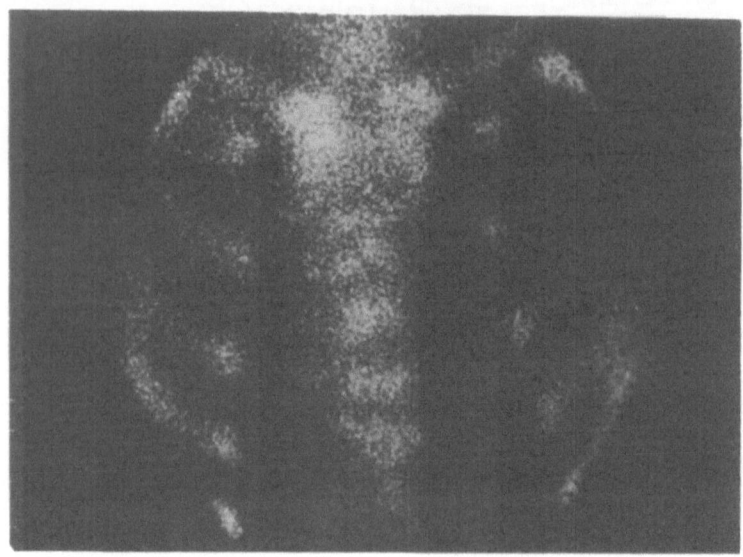

Figure 5. Bone scan of anterior thorax with 'beading' of costochondral junctions.

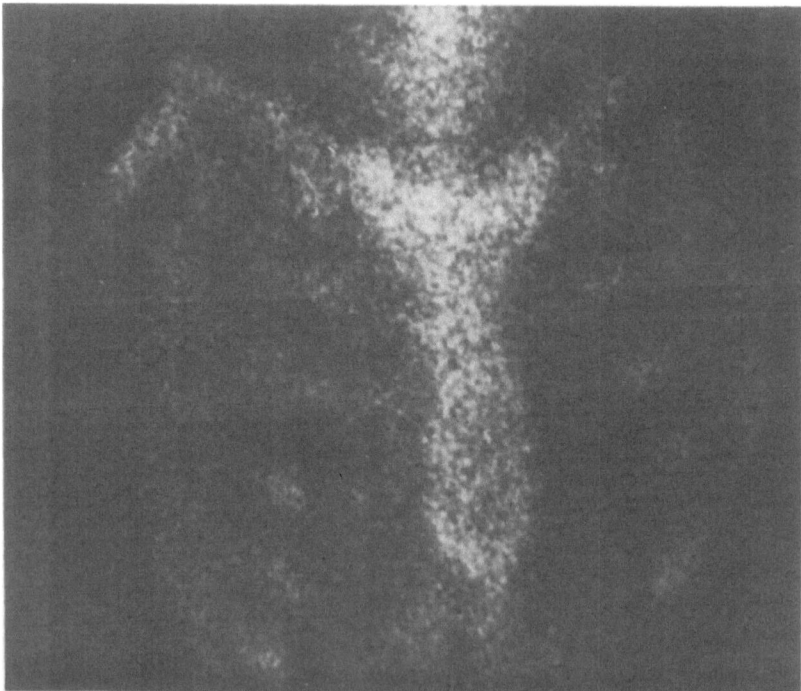

Figure 6. Bone scan of anterior thorax with increased tracer uptake by the sternum particularly at lateral borders – the "tie" sternum.

1.1. *Osteoporosis*

In osteoporosis there is usually only a very gradual change in bone mass that occurs over many years and in accord with this the bone scan appearances are usually normal. Occasionally, very poor scan images with low bone to background ratios are noted in severe osteoporosis and it has been suggested that these occur in severe or "end-stage" osteoporosis because of markedly reduced or absent osteoblastic axtivity (10). Osteoporotic bones are abnormally brittle and pathologic fractures may occur. These appear on the bone scan as focal areas of increased tracer uptake and where vertebral collapse has occurred the scan appearances are characteristic. Isotope activity in the spine is generally reduced but there is linear increased tracer uptake corresponding to the whole of any collapsed vertebral body or bodies (Figure 7). This increased uptake usually fades within a year following vertebral collapse (11) and the bone scan may, therefore, be of value in assessing the interval since fracture has occurred.

1.2. *Osteomalacia*

The bone scan appearances in osteomalacia are usually strongly suggestive of the presence of a metabolic bone disorder (8). However, the scan features are non-specific and may be seen in other metabolic bone disorders (e.g. renal osteodystrophy). All the features listed in Table 1 may be observed and when pseudofractures are present these are seen on the bone scan as focal areas of increased tracer uptake (12) (Figure 8). Conventional radiographs of the ribs may be normal and in this situation bone scanning is the more sensitive investigation (12). Pseudofractures in the pelvis may occasionally be missed on the bone scan, due either to their symmetrical nature or because they are obscured by bladder activity (8).

Table 1. Metabolic features on bone scan.

1. Increased tracer uptake in axial skeleton.
2. Increased tracer uptake in long bones.
3. Increased tracer uptake in periarticular areas (wrist).
4. Prominent calvarium and mandible.
5. Beading of the costo-chondral junctions.
6. "Tie" sternum.
7. Faint or absent kidney images.

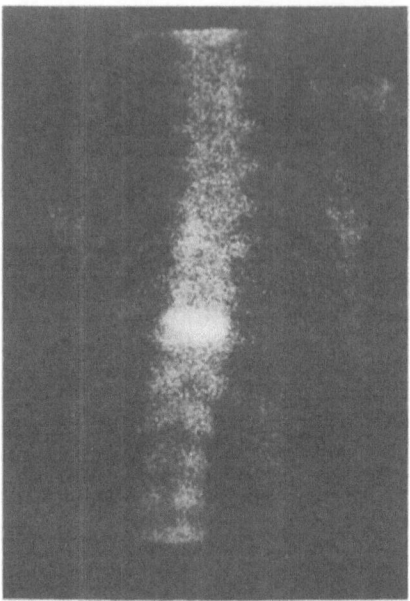

Figure 7. Linearly increased tracer uptake corresponding to a collapsed vertebral body in the spine of an osteoporotic patient. (Reproduced with permission from the Editor of the Scottish medical Journal).

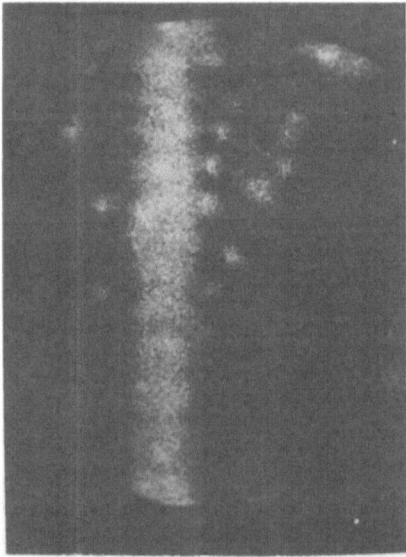

Figure 8. Multiple focal abnormalities representing pseudofractures are seen in the ribs of an osteomalacic patient.

1.3. *Renal osteodystrophy*

Renal osteodystrophy produces the most striking bone scans seen in the various metabolic bone diseases. It is thought that most of the abnormal bone scan findings are due to the effect of secondary hyperparathyroidism, but co-existing osteomalacia probably contributes. Typical bone scan appearances are of markedly increased tracer uptake throughout the axial and peripheral skeleton (6, 13, 14). In keeping with this the kidneys are frequently not visualised. The calvarium and mandible appear particularly prominent and beading of the costo-chondral junctions and a "tie" sternum are also commonly seen. Osteosclerosis is occasionally seen in radiographs of the spine in patients with renal osteodystrophy (the so called "rugger jersey spine"). The bone scan equivalent of this is linear areas of slightly increased tracer uptake against a background of generalised high uptake in the spine (15).

1.4. *Primary hyperparathyroidism*

Patients with primary hyperparathyroidism can have bone scans ranging from normal to appearances similar to those found in renal osteodystrophy depending on the severity of skeletal involvement (5, 7). Focal hot spots are uncommon but may be due to vertebral collapse, ectopic calcification (16) or bone cysts (17).

2. BONE SCANNING COMPARED WITH RADIOLOGY IN METABOLIC BONE DISEASE

We have evaluated bone scans and radiological skeletal surveys in 80 patients with various metabolic bone disorders (27 with osteoporosis, 14 with primary hyperparathyroidism, 24 with renal osteodystrophy and 15 with osteomalacia) (11) (Table 2). It was shown that in the osteoporotic group radiology is the investigation of choice but the bone scan may be of value in assessing the interval since vertebral collapse and perhaps in alerting an observer to the presence of an underlying condition which may be responsible for accelerated bone loss e.g. primary hyperparathyroidism or thyrotoxicosis. In the other patient groups the bone scan was found to be the more sensitive investigation and we believe it should be performed prior to x-ray. In our study, patients with renal osteodystrophy and osteomalacia were severe examples of disease and one would not expect the bone scan to be abnormal in 100% of

106

Table 2. Comparison of X-ray and scan sensitivity in metabolic bone disease.

Disease	X-Ray	Scan
Osteoporosis	81%	0% (41%) [a]
Primary Hyperparathyroidism	21%	50%
Renal Osteodystrophy	58%	100%
Osteomalacia	60%	100%

[a] If the non-metabolic bone scan feature of vertebral collapse (which would suggest the presence of osteoporosis) is included then sensitivity rises to 41%.

Source: from Fogelman and Carr, (11) by permission of the Editor of Clinical Radiology.

cases (Table 2) when 'milder' disease was studied. Nevertheless in this selected population the bone scan undoubtedly proved superior to conventional radiology.

While the bone scan is relatively non-specific and x-rays may on occasion show specific changes, e.g. sub-periosteal resorption in hyperparathyroidism, it is likely that if the bone scan does not suggest the presence of a metabolic bone disorder then radiology will also be negative.

3. SEMI-QUANTITATIVE EVALUATION OF THE BONE SCAN IMAGE (the Metabolic Index)

It is possible to derive a semi-quantitative diagnostic index for metabolic bone disease from the bone scan. We have numerically graded each of the 7 features listed in Table 1 on a scale 0–normal, 1–abnormal or 2–markedly abnormal, and have defined the total score as the Metabolic Index (9). Using this scoring system we have shown that it is possible to differentiate groups of patients with osteomalacia, renal osteodystrophy, primary hyperparathyroidism, acromegaly and osteoporosis from a control population. There was, however, overlap of individual patient results with the control range and as one might expect this was most marked in the osteoporosis group (9).

The bone scan may, therefore, be of considerable value in the assessment of patients with metabolic bone disease but unfortunately is least likely to be of assistance in those patients providing the most difficulty in clinical practice – e.g. patients with osteoporosis, 'mild' primary hyperparathyroidism or subclinical osteomalacia often have normal bone scans. It is in such cases that accurate quantitation of skeletal uptake of radiopharmaceutical would be of value.

4. QUANTITATION OF SKELETAL UPTAKE OF RADIOPHARMACEUTICAL

Simple quantitation of skeletal tracer uptake can be obtained from a bone scan image by measuring the bone to soft tissue (B/ST) ratio (7, 14). However, this is a relatively crude technique where a small area of bone is selected which may not reflect a small yet significant change in the total skeletal uptake of radiopharmaceutical. There is also the problem of standardizing the 'soft-tissue' since counts per unit area vary with vascularity and muscle bulk. We have found that there is considerable overlap of B/ST measurements in disease patients and a control population (8, 18) and therefore believe that this technique is of little value in clinical practice.

In order to quantify total skeletal uptake of tracer accurately, we measure the 24 hour whole body retention (WBR) of technetium diphosphonate using a shadow-shield whole body monitor (18). We have shown that this method is sensitive in the detection of patients with increased bone turnover and that patients with Paget's disease, osteomalacia, primary hyperparathyroidism and renal osteodystrophy can be clearly differentiated from a control population (Figure 9).

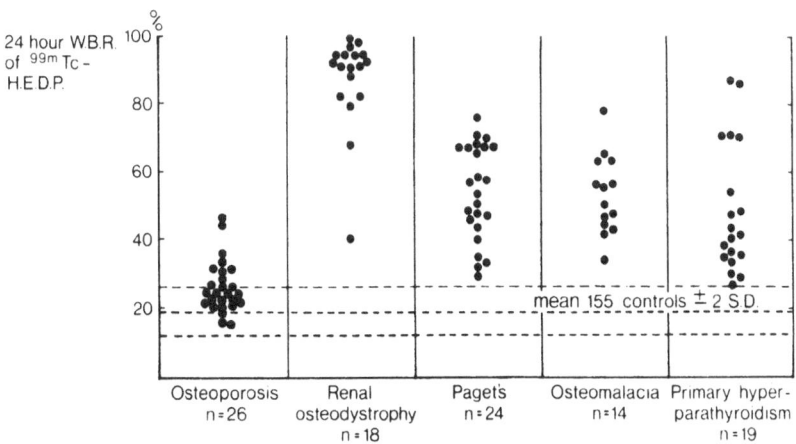

Figure 9. Results of WBR studies in individual patients with metabolic bone disease.

Note that each individual patient result in these groups lies outwith the control range. Most patients with osteoporosis have normal values for WBR although approximately one third of the subjects that we have studied were found to have elevated values. In this group transilial bone biopsies have been performed and it is of interest that those patients with elevated values for WBR have histological evidence of increased bone turnover. It is possible that this test may eventually allow us to identify a sub-population of women who shortly after the menopause are passing through a period of accelerated bone loss and who may, therefore, be at risk of subsequently developing osteoporosis. In a recent study in patients with primary hyperparathyroidism we have shown a good correlation between WBR and plasma parathyroid hormone ($r = 0.86$, $p < 0.001$) and a moderate correlation with serum alkaline phosphatase values ($r = 0.58$, $p < 0.05$). Also repeat studies of WBR performed in 5 patients pre and post-parathyroidectomy have shown a fall from elevated to normal or near normal values in all cases (19).

The results from these studies suggest that WBR provides a sensitive measure of skeletal metabolism and we would anticipate that this technique will find widespread application in clinical practice. Whole body retention also has potential application as a screening procedure in patients with recurrent renal stones, for they are known to have an above average incidence of primary hyperparathyroidism. Patients who have had previous gastric surgery, those on long term anti-convulsant therapy and elderly women who fracture a femur could be screened for osteomalacia.

The skeleton is a difficult organ to investigate and currently there is no satisfactory technique for assessing skeletal metabolic activity. Whole body retention of technetium diphosphonate provides a sensitive means of detecting increased bone turnover and it is likely that this tracer technique combined with routine bone scan imaging will increasingly be used to assess the living, metabolically active skeleton.

REFERENCES

1. Edelstyn GA, Gillespie PJ, Crebbell FS: The radiological demonstration of osseous metastases: experimental observations. Clin Radiol 18:158-162, 1967.
2. Jones AG, Francis MD, Davis MA: Bone scanning: radionuclide reaction mechanisms. Semin Nucl Med 6:3-18, 1976.
3. Tofe AJ, Francis MD, Harvey WJ: Correlation of neoplasm with incidence and localisation of skeletal metastases: an analysis of 1355 diphosphonate bone scans. J Nucl Med 16:986-989, 1975.
4. Citrin DL, Bessent RG, Greig WR: A comparison of the sensitivity and accuracy of the 99m-Tc-phosphate bone scan and skeletal radiography in the diagnosis of bone metastases. Clin Radiol 28:107-117, 1977.

5. Sy WM: Bone scan in primary hyperparathyroidism. J Nucl Med 15:1089-1091, 1974.

6. Sy WM, Mittal AK: Bone scan in chronic dialysis patients with evidence of secondary hyperparathyroidism and renal osteodystrophy. Br J Radiol 48:878-884, 1975.

7. Wiegmann T, Rosenthall L, Kaye M: Technetium 99m-pyrophosphate bone scans in hyperparathyroidism. J Nucl Med 18:231-235, 1977.

8. Fogelman I, McKillop JH, Bessent RG, Boyle IT, Turner JG, Greig WR: The role of bone scanning in osteomalacia. J Nucl Med 19:245-248, 1978.

9. Fogelman I, Citrin DL, Turner JG, Hay ID, Bessent RG, Boyle IT: Semi-quantitative interpretation of the bone scan in metabolic bone disease. Eur J Nucl Med 4:287-289, 1979.

10. Levine SB, Haines JE, Larson SM, Andrews TM: Reduced skeletal localisation of 99m Tc-diphosphonate in two cases of severe osteoporosis. Clin Nucl Med 2:318-321, 1977.

11. Fogelman I, Carr D: A comparison of bone scanning and radiology in the evaluation of patients with metabolic bone disease. Clin Radiol 31:321-326, 1980.

12. Fogelman I, McKillop JH, Greig WR, Boyle IT: Pseudo-fractures of the ribs detected by bone scanning. J Nucl Med 18:1236-1237, 1977.

13. Olgaard K, Heerfordt J, Madsen S: Scintigraphic skeletal changes in uremic patients on regular haemodialysis. Nephron 17:325-334, 1976.

14. Lien JW, Wiegmann T, Rosenthall L, Kaye M: Abnormal 99m Technetium-tin-pyrophosphate bone scans in chronic renal failure. Clin Nephrol 6:509-512, 1976.

15. Fogelman I, Citrin DL: Bone scanning in metabolic bone disease: A review. Applied Radiology, in press.

16. Sy WM, Mottola O, Lao RS, Smith A, Freund HR: Unusual bone images in hyperparathyroidism. Br J Radiol 50:740-744, 1977.

17. Evens RG, Ashburn W, Bartter FC: Strontium 85 scanning of a "brown tumour" in a patient with parathyroid carcinoma. Br J Radiol 42:224-225, 1969.

18. Fogelman I, Bessent RG, Turner JG, Citrin DL, Boyle IT, Greig WR: The use of whole-body retention of Tc-99m diphosphonate in the diagnosis of metabolic bone disease. J Nucl Med 19:270-275, 1978.

19. Fogelman I, Bessent RG, Beastall G, Boyle IT: Estimation of skeletal involvement in primary hyperparathyroidism: use of 24-hour whole-body retention of technetium-99m diphosphonate. Ann Int Med 92:65-67, 1980.

9. QUANTITATIVE BONE SCINTIGRAPHY IN RENAL OSTEODYSTROPHY

PIETER DE GRAAF

Quantitative bone scintigraphy
Bone scintigraphy in hemodialysis patients
Uptake mechanism in renal bone disorders

1. INTRODUCTION

1.1. *Renal osteodystrophy*

In renal failure, a disturbance in the conversion in the kidney of vitamin D into a hormonal form essential for the mobilization of calcium from both intestine and bone (1) and a disturbance in renal phosphate excretion leading to phosphate retention (2), are the two major mechanisms involved in the pathogenesis of renal bone disease. Both mechanisms cause hypocalcemia and, subsequently, hyperparathyroidism. Since the production of active vitamin D metabolites is diminished or absent in advanced renal failure, the intestinal absorption of calcium will be blunted and the skeletal response to the calcemic action of parathyroid hormone (PTH) will be reduced.

Consequently, a greater amount of PTH will be required to mobilize calcium from bone and the skeleton will continually be sacrificed in an attempt to maintain serum calcium within the normal range. This secondary hyperparathyroidism will cause an increase in the turnover and resorption of bone (osteitis fibrosa) while the calcium and active vitamin D metabolite deficiencies will result in defective mineralization of bone (osteomalacia). These bone abnormalities, which may be associated with either an overall deficit of bone (osteoporosis) or, less common, bone excess (osteosclerosis), are collectively termed renal osteodystrophy.

In the course of progressive renal failure, the effects of hyperparathyroidism on bone generally precede those of defective mineralization but both components of renal osteodystrophy are usually present in patients on maintenance hemodialysis (3). Symptomatic bone disease, however,

Pauwels EKJ, Schütte HE, Taconis WK, eds, Bone scintigraphy, p 111–125.
Copyright © 1981 Martinus Nijhoff Publishers bv, The Hague/Boston/London. All rights reserved.

is relatively uncommon and usually occurs late in the course of renal failure but when present, it is difficult to manage conservatively. This stresses the importance of the early diagnosis and treatment of bone disease in renal failure.

1.2. *Routine diagnostic procedures*

Biochemical data, i.e. serum calcium, phosphate, alkaline phosphatase and iPTH, may provide information about the presence and the nature of renal bone disease but, in itself, the value of biochemical analysis is limited. Radiographic techniques are also not highly sensitive for the detection of renal osteodystrophy, in particular osteomalacia, even when sensitive magnification techniques are used (4). Thus, accurate diagnosis of renal osteodystrophy depends on the histologic examination of bone, which is usually obtained from the iliac crest. Undecalcified stained thin bone sections can then be evaluated by qualitative or quantitative (morphometric) analysis to assess the degree of bone formation, resorption and mineralization. Bone microscopy, however, does not necessarily inform about the state of involvement of the whole skeleton and bone biopsies cannot be repeated often. The invasive nature of this technique, as well as the frequent absence of radiographic abnormalities, probably contributed to the growing interest in the efficacy of bone scintigraphy in the diagnosis of renal osteodystrophy.

1.3. *Bone scintigraphy*

In recent years, bone scintigraphy has been recognized as a sensitive method, superior to radiographic skeletal analysis, for the early detection and assessment of the severity of renal osteodystrophy (5–12). A chief limitation of this method, however, is the inability to distinguish which of the two major components of renal bone disease, i.e. secondary hyperparathyroidism and osteomalacia, is the main cause of the increased skeletal radiotracer uptake. This is subject of controversy, (5, 6, 8, 12) since the mechanism of radiotracer uptake in bone is not precisely known (13) and quantitative studies correlating bone radiotracer uptake with bone morphometry have not been performed in renal osteodystrophy.

Apart from the nonspecificity of the results obtained, technical problems, such as those resulting from increased soft-tissue activity due to impaired renal radiotracer excretion (14), further limit the application of qualitative bone scintigraphy in patients with renal failure. With the exception of patients with severe renal bone disease whereby so-called "superscans" are obtained, increased soft-tissue activity results in diminished bone-to-soft-tissue contrast which may markedly lower the quality of the scan. Also, the radioactivity retained in the body complicates the quantitative evaluation of skeletal radiotracer uptake in renal osteodystrophy and its comparison with that in normal bone. Possibly for this reason, detailed quantitative scintigraphic skeletal analysis has not been performed in patients with renal failure and quantitative studies in such patients have been limited to bone-to-soft-tissue activity ratios in the distal femur (6, 8) and whole body radionuclide retention at 24 hours (15).

The need for noninvasive sensitive techniques for the diagnosis and follow-up of metabolic bone disease in dialysis patients has stimulated our interest in the efficacy of more detailed quantitative bone scintigraphy. Using hemodialysis to reduce elevated soft-tissue activity at scintigraphy, an attempt was made to assess the diagnostic sensitivity of quantitative bone scintigraphy as compared to qualitative bone scintigraphic, biochemical, radiographic and bone histologic studies. The second aim of these studies was to determine if one of the two major components of renal osteodystrophy is a major determinant for skeletal radiotracer uptake. Our clinical observations on the efficacy and possible specificity of quantitative bone scintigraphy in the diagnosis and follow-up during treatment of renal osteodystrophy are presented briefly in this chapter.

2. TECHNIQUES OF HEMODIALYSIS AND QUANTITATIVE BONE SCINTIGRAPHY

2.1. *Hemodialysis before scintigraphy*

In initial studies in virtually untreated dialysis patients (9, 16) we found that, when the patients were dialyzed from 15 minutes to 5 hours after i.v. administration of 10 mCi Tc-99m EHDP per 70 kg bodyweight, the circulating radioactivity at scintigraphy after 6 hours could be reduced to $7 \pm 3\%$ (mean $\pm$SD) of the initial peak circulating activity measured. These mean radioactivity levels were only slightly higher than those found for 8 normals ($5 \pm 2\%$). A parallel-plate (RP6 HP, acrylonitrite membrane) artificial kidney was used throughout. Initially, the artificial kidney was connected to a so-called single-patient unit to avoid radioactive contamination of the central bathing-water system. This device, however, had to be abandoned since the use of recirculating dialysate was found to cause free pertechnetate formation; its secretion by the stomach, which occured in the absence of thyroid imaging, suggested gastric calcification (17).

The initial reduction of the soft-tissue activity to (near) normal levels at scintigraphy, however, resulted in part from increased uptake of the tracer in the diseased skeleton and, in later studies, it became apparent that hemodialysis reduced, but failed to normalize, circulating radioactivity in patients with only minimal bone disease after treatment (18). This problem has not yet been solved, partly because the nature of our studies is such that repeated examination of these patients is not feasible since they are also frequently subjected to other radiodiagnostic procedures. Incidental observations suggest that the problem of elevated circulating activity, when present, is not solved by using methylene diphosphonate (MDP), which has a slightly more rapid blood clearance rate than EHDP (19). Also, the use of other types of artificial kidneys did not yield a greater reduction of the soft-tissue activity than the parallel-plate kidney used. No evidence could be found to show that this increased circulating activity contributes significantly to the results of the quantitative scintigraphic analysis (16). However, since its influence could not be assessed accurately the quantitative values obtained for patients with minimal bone disease may in fact be slightly lower than presented.

2.2. Quantification of skeletal radiotracer uptake without computer assistance

Scintigraphy was performed after 6 hours with a large-field gamma camera provided with two scalers and controls to register counts in selected regions of interest. Images were obtained by standard positioning of all skeletal parts under the detector. The quantitative data were collected by calculating count rates within standardized selected regions of the skeleton (including soft-tissues) and were expressed as kC/sec., dose-corrected for 10 mCi-99m.

Bladder activity, if present, was taken into account. The kilocounts (kC) of radioactivity registered in these regions were: head region, 200 kC; chest region, 300 kC; spine, 80 kC; pelvic region, 350 kC; hip region, 250 kC; thighs, 75 kC; knee regions, 75 kC; lower legs, 50 kC; ankles and feet, 25 kC; and hands, 25 kC. The activity in the lower extremities was registered separately. The sum of the activity rates was used as an index of the total skeletal activity (TSA) and was expressed as kC/sec/10 mCi. Normal values (2.6–4.1, mean 3.4) were obtained from 10 age-matched controls.

2.3. *Quantification of skeletal radiotracer uptake with computer assistance*

All gamma camera data were recorded on magnetic disks with the aid of a dedicated minicomputer for later quantitative analysis. The preset time for computer imaging was 120 sec. The standardized regions of the skeleton were selected for quantitative analysis using a cursor (Figure 1). This has the obvious advantages of eliminating more soft-tissue activity and thus providing a more detailed and precise skeletal analysis of radiotracer uptake. The count rates within these flagged sites were calculated by the computer and expressed as kC/sec/10 mCi. To minimize observer errors, the mean number of counts per channel in these areas was calculated as well and expressed as C/sec/Ch/10 mCi. The number of counts per channel in the iliac crest bone biopsy site was measured; the bone biopsies were taken shortly hereafter. Because of the relatively small region of interest, the mean of the number of counts per channel of three consecutive measurements was calculated and expressed as C/sec/Ch/10 mCi. The sum of the activity in all flagged regions of interest was also used as an index of the total skeletal activity (TSA). The sum of the number of counts per channel in these areas was expressed as the total counts per channel. Normal values for the three computer-assisted scintigraphic methods were obtained from another 10 age-matched controls.

3. SENSITIVITY OF QUANTITATIVE BONE SCINTIGRAPHY VERSUS OTHER DIAGNOSTIC PROCEDURES

3.1. *Bone scintigraphy without computer assistance*

Quantitative bone scintigraphy was initially performed in 30 chronic dialysis patients (9). All patients showed histologic evidence of renal osteodystrophy. Alkaline phosphatase values were elevated in 23 patients (76%) but radiographic abnormalities were found in only 14 patients (46%); this low incidence of radiographic abnormalities illustrates the insensitivity of this technique with respect to skeletal lesions in renal osteodystrophy. In contrast, 25 patients (83%) showed bone scan abnormalities. The quantitative scintigraphic analysis, however,

116

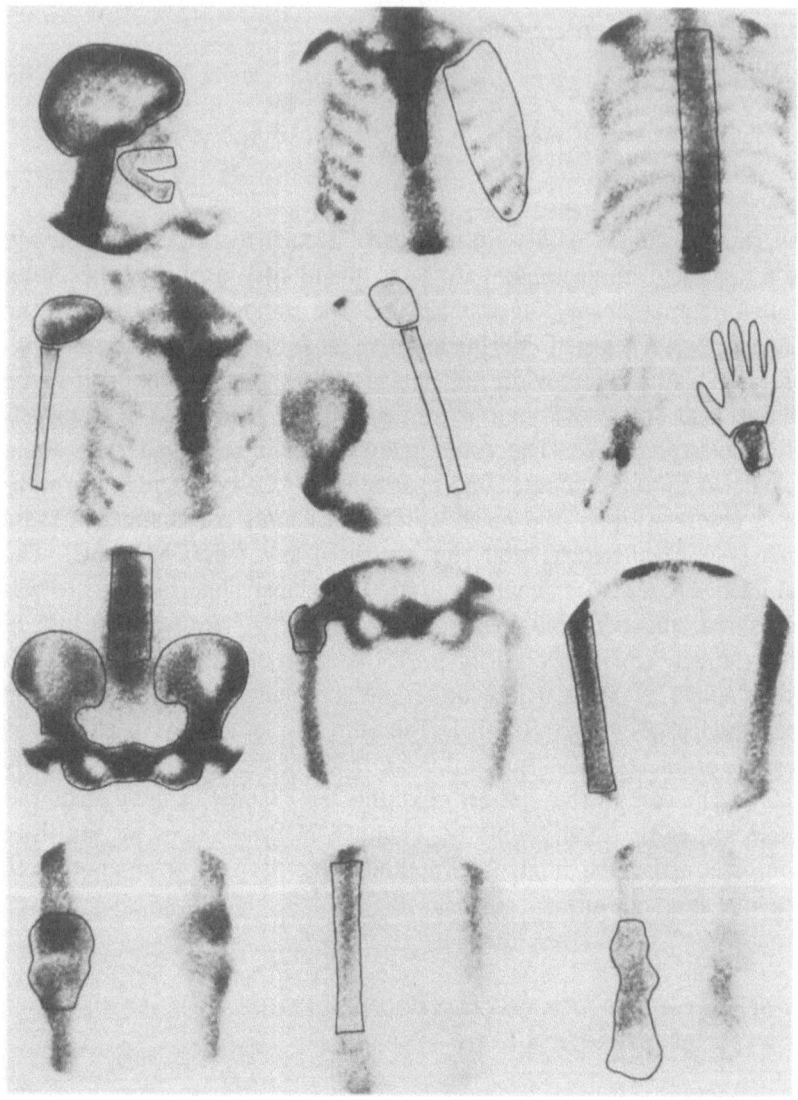

Figure 1. Bone scan of a dialysis patient showing the light-pen flagged regions of the skeleton selected for computer evaluation of radiotracer uptake.

showed an often markedly elevated TSA (range 5.72–11.38 kC/sec/10 mCi) in all patients when compared with the normals. Similar results were obtained in a second study performed in 35 patients, in which iPTH results were included (20). With the exception of the patient with the lowest TSA (4.58 kC/sec/10 mCi), who showed histologic signs of only osteomalacia, all patients had some histologic features of both osteitis fibrosa and osteomalacia. Whereas alkaline phosphatase and iPTH exceeded the maximum normal values in only 21 and 19 patients, respectively, the TSA was elevated in all patients (range 4.58–10.77 kC/sec/ 10 mCi). Even though an – generally mild – increase in soft-tissue activity occurred in several patients with minimal bone disease (which contributed to the quantitative data obtained) the quantitative analysis clearly separated the vast majority of the patients with histologically proven renal osteodystrophy from normals. Although the precise influence of the elevated soft-tissue activity, when present, on the quantitative data could not be determined, several observations indicate that this elevated soft-tissue activity does not contribute to the quantitative skeletal data to a major extent. Quantitative bone scintigraphy, performed in at present two patients with acute renal failure and a normal skeleton, showed that the TSA (after prior hemodialysis) exceeded the normal range (2.6–4.1 kC/sec) by a maximum of 1 kC/sec. Assuming that the upper limit of the normal range would be 5.1 kC/sec. i.e. taking the maximum of elevated soft-tissue activity into account, the TSA for over 90% of our chronic dialysis patients studied exceeded this value as well. Furthermore, if the dialysis patients studied demonstrated elevated soft-tissue activity at scintigraphy, the TSA was relatively low as compared to patients with normal or low circulating activity, who generally showed a markedly increase in the TSA. Quantitative bone scintigraphy, performed in 15 patients with recent renal transplants and good graft function (mean ±SD serum creatinine 98±23 μmol/l), demonstrated an elevated TSA in 14 of these patients in the absence of elevated soft-tissue activity (16). These data also indicate that the quantitative results obtained in patients with renal bone disease are predominantly governed by the degree of skeletal pathology.

3.2. *Bone scintigraphy with computer assistance*

When computer analysis became available in our department, the quantitative scintigraphic studies were repeated in 30 dialysis patients with and without the aid of the computer, as described above. The biochemical values for these patients were generally within the normal – or near normal – range as a result of surgical and/or intensive medical treatment for a period of at least six months before this study (18). However, histologic features of hyperparathyroidism and osteomalacia, although often mild, were still present in the bone biopsy specimens of 97% and 100% of these patients, respectively.

118

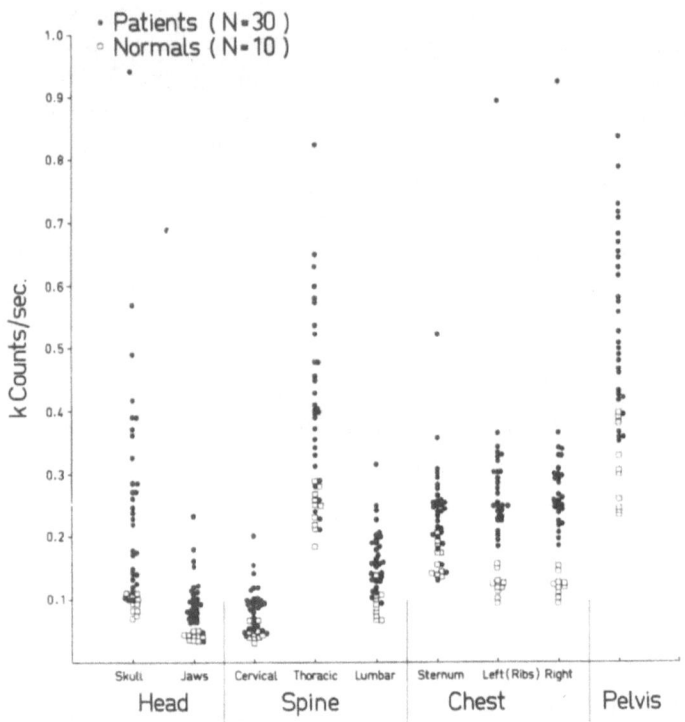

a

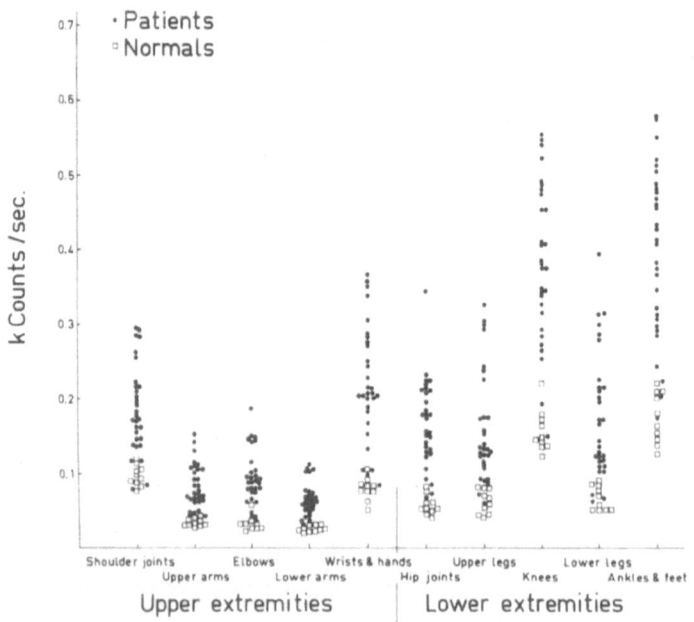

b

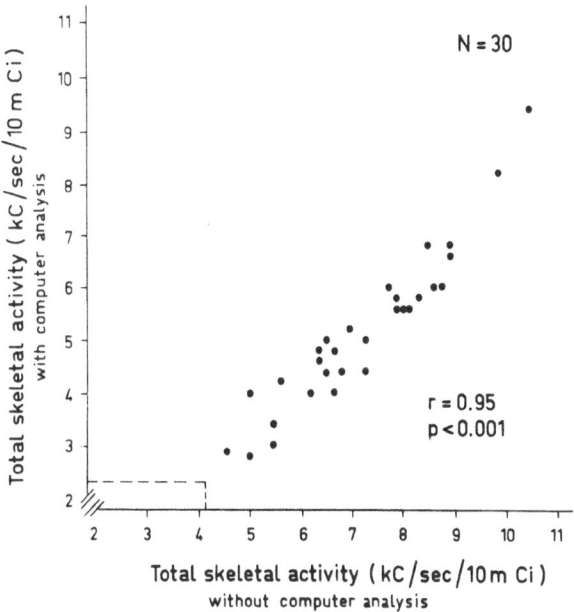

Figure 3. Relationship between the total skeletal activities assessed with and without computer. Dotted lines represent upper limits of normal values for both methods.

The quantitative scintigraphic data, obtained with the computer in the flagged areas of the skeleton (Figure 1), were elevated in the majority of the patients (Figure 2) but the TSA, assessed with and without computer assistance (Figure 3), as well as the total counts per channel, again exceeded the maximum normal values in all cases. The fact that the measurements performed without the computer included more bone and soft-tissue activity explains why the TSA thus obtained for patients as well as normals was higher than that found with computer evaluation (Figure 3). As expected, the correlation between the results of the two methods was highly significant (Figure 3). Also, the total counts per channel in the flagged skeletal sites showed a highly significant relationship with the computer-assessed TSA and the noncomputer-assessed TSA ($p < 0.001$). Furthermore, the number of counts per channel at the bone biopsy sites correlated significantly ($p < 0.001$) with both the TSA and the total counts per channel which indicates that increased radio-

←

Figure 2. Quantitative data obtained with the computer within the flagged regions of interest in patients and normals, expressed as kC/sec corrected for 10 mCi ^{99m}Tc EHDP dose.

tracer uptake in the whole skeleton may generally be considered to be representative of that in the iliac crest bone of patients with renal bone disease.

The quantitative scintigraphic methods used were probably able to distinguish all patients with histologically abnormal bone from normals. This suggests that computer evaluation of skeletal radiotracer uptake, when performed after lowering soft-tissue activity by hemodialysis, provides a fairly reliable and detailed method for detecting the presence and severity of renal osteodystrophy in dialysis patients. This technique is more sensitive than biochemical and radiographic methods and neither the costs nor the radiation dose exceeds that of radiographic skeletal analysis.

Thus, the use of scintigraphy for the routine detection and follow-up of renal osteodystrophy in dialysis patients may reduce the need for repeated bone biopsies or provide additional information since it informs about the extent of osteodystrophy in the whole skeleton. The dialysis method, however, needs perfecting to improve the bone image quality and the accuracy of the quantitative skeletal analysis in patients with only minimal renal osteodystrophy.

4. INTERPRETATION OF INCREASED SKELETAL RADIOTRACER UPTAKE IN RENAL OSTEODYSTROPHY

4.1. *Factors influencing radiotracer uptake in bone*

In normal bone, the uptake of Tc-99m labeled phosphorous agents is thought to result primarily from binding to the inorganic constituents of bone, i.e. from adsorption on calcium phosphate, present either as hydroxyapatite crystals or as small nuclei of calcium phosphate at mineralization sites, a precess referred to as "chemisorption" (21, 22). Microautoradiographic studies (21, 23, 24) support the view that the tracer does not bind directly to the osteoid tissue but to the bone matrix where mineralization occurs, in the proximity of sites of osteoblastic activity. However, since these areas are located at the interface of osteoid and mineralized bone, some binding to the organic matrix cannot be excluded. Proposed factors affecting an increase of the tracer uptake in bone include a high rate of bone (mineral) turnover, which is known to be associated with large surface areas for exchange and adsorption (21, 22), increased local vascularity (25), high enzyme activity (26) and binding to increased amounts of organic bone, in particular the immature collagen (27).

Increased amounts of amorphous calcium phosphate have been demonstrated in areas of rapid metabolic bone activity in various states and these amorphous calcium phosphates, which are of low density and high hydration, in particular appear to absorb the radiotracer (22). Appreciable binding of the Tc-99m labeled bone-seeking agents on excess organic bone matrix, however, has recently been questioned and is considered unlikely unless the organic matrix is nucleated with calcium phosphate (22). Also, the evidence that tracer uptake is influenced by enzymatic receptor binding is at present not considered conclusive (22). Furthermore, increased vascularity does not appear to be a major factor in tracer uptake either (28).

An increased rate of bone turnover, high enzyme activity and an increased formation of – defectively mineralized – organic bone coexists in renal osteodystrophy. Although all of these factors could contribute to the increased skeletal radiotracer uptake in this condition, the data mentioned above suggest that this increased uptake is probably determined primarily by the degree of bone turnover, rather than by an excess amount of organic bone. Thus, the effects of hyperparathyroidism on bone might prove to be a more important cause of the increased tracer uptake in renal osteodystrophy than the degree of osteomalacia. Our clinical observations in this respect support this view.

4.2. Relationship between quantitative (noncomputer-assessed) scintigraphic data and biochemical and bone histologic data before treatment

In our initial study (9), significant relationships (p < 0.001) were found between the TSA and alkaline phosphatase as well as the histologic (semi-quantitatively assessed) degree of osteitis fibrosa. The relationship between the TSA and the histologic degree of osteomalacia was of low significance (0.05 < p < 0.10). These findings suggested that the effects of hyperparathyroidism on bone are a major determinant for increased tracer uptake in renal osteodystrophy and marked parathyroid hyperplasia was subsequently confirmed in 10 patients with a high TSA who underwent parathyroidectomy hereafter. The observation that the TSA had not decreased several weeks after parathyroidectomy suggested that PTH in itself does not have a direct effect on the tracer uptake in bone.

The hypothesis that the degree of hyperparathyroidism is a more important factor in tracer uptake than is the degree of osteomalacia, was further investigated by correlating the results of quantitative bone scintigraphy, performed in 35 patients who had not yet been subjected to parathyroidectomy, with those of biochemical and quantitative bone histologic (morphometric) studies (20). A significant relationship (p < 0.001) was found between the biochemical parameters of hyperparathyroidism, i.e. alkaline phosphatase and iPTH, and the histologic parameters, i.e. the osteoblast surface, osteoclast count, degree of fibrosis and the degree of endosteal cells lining the bone surface. The relationship between the TSA and all of these parameters of hyperparathyroidism was statistically highly significant (P < 0.001) but the relationships between the TSA and the osteoid volume and osteoid surface were statistically of lesser significance (p < 0.05) and, in addition, could have been positively influenced by the increased amounts of osteoid accompanying increased bone turnover. These findings further suggested that increased bone turnover, rather than the amount of (osteomalacic) osteoid, is the major cause of the increased skeletal radiotracer uptake in renal osteodystrophy.

4.3. *Relationship between changes in the quantitative (noncomputerassessed) scintigraphic data and biochemical and bone histologic data during treatment*

Further support for this view was obtained when statistically significant correlations were found between the changes in the TSA and the changes in the biochemical and histologic parameters of hyperparathyroidism during treatment of renal osteodystrophy; the changes in the TSA did not correlate with the changes in osteoid excess. In this study (18) the TSA improved in 22 out of 25 patients but did not normalize in any of these cases, including 5 patients who received a well-functioning renal transplant. For the other 20 patients studied, subtotal parathyroidectomy (11 patients) or medical treatment (9 patients) led to a reduction in the histologic degree of hyperparathyroidism in 17 of the 19 patients in whom bone histologic evaluation could be performed. Osteoid excess was reduced in 13 patients, but an improvement in the degree of osteomalacic osteoid occurred in only 4 of the 19 patients. The changes in the TSA, with one exception, parallelled the changes in the histologic features of hyperparathyroidism, irrespective of the changes in the osteoid excess. These findings suggested that for the evaluation of treatment of renal osteodystrophy, bone scintigraphy provides information primarily about the changes in the degree of hyperparathyroidism.

4.4. Relationship between quantitative (computer-assessed) data and bone histologic data after treatment

The scintigraphic studies performed after treatment with the aid of a computer in the 30 patients mentioned above (3.2) again demonstrated significant correlations between the results of the various scintigraphic methods used and the histologic features of hyperparathyroidism, but not with the amount of (osteomalacic) osteoid. Interestingly, the correlations between the scintigraphic results and the osteoblastic and osteoclastic activity increased in significance with the probable specificity of the scintigraphic method used, i.e. the TSA, the sum of the counts per channel and the counts per channel in the biopsy area, respectively. The observation that the accumulated radioactivity measured at the bone biopsy site showed a significant relationship ($p < 0.001$) with the TSA, which indicates that the uptake of the tracer in the whole skeleton is probably representative of that in the iliac crest, supports the validity of our studies correlating the TSA with iliac crest bone pathology in patients with renal osteodystrophy.

4.5. Concluding remarks

Although our observations do not contribute to the knowledge concerning the mechanism of radiotracer uptake in renal osteodystrophy, the data presented suggest that this – often markedly – increased uptake is dependant mainly on the degree of bone turnover and cellular, in particular osteoblastic, activity. Thus, hyperparathyroidism, rather than the amount of (osteomalacic) osteoid *per se* (8) appears to be the major cause of increased tracer uptake in renal osteodystrophy. Similar conclusions, based on the bone scan patterns, have previously been reported by others (5, 11).

Although bone turnover is governed by the degree of hyperparathyroidism, PTH in itself probably has no significant direct effect on tracer uptake in bone. Also, the product of the osteoblasts, i.e. the amount of osteoid, does not appear to determine the uptake of radiotracer to any considerable extent. As in various other states of rapid metabolic bone activity (21, 22), this increased uptake probably occurs in the proximity of sites of osteoblastic activity. Possibly, increased bone (mineral) turnover in association with defective maturation of amorphous calcium phosphate to its crystalline phase, results in an increased amount of amorphous calcium phosphate in renal osteodystrophy as well. These amorphous calcium phosphates might cumulate and be distributed diffusely through bone, similar to the patchy, irregular distribution of newly formed bone by the osteoblasts, thereby providing increased surface areas for radiotracer bone binding. Further arguments to support this hypothesis, however, could not be obtained.

REFERENCES

1. DeLuca HF: Vitamin D metabolism and function. Arch Int Med 138:836-847, 1978.
2. Slatopolsky E, Rutherford E, Hruska K, Martin K, Klahr S: How important is phosphate in the pathogenesis of renal osteodystrophy? Arch Int Med 138:848-852, 1978.
3. Alvarez-Ude F, Feest TG, Ward MK, Pierides AM, Ellis HA, Peart KM, Simpson W, Weightman D, Kerr DNS: Hemodialysis bone disease: Correlation between clinical histologic and other findings. Kidney Int 14:68-73, 1978.
4. Ritz E, Prager P, Krempien B, Bommer J, Malluche HH, Schmidt-Gayk H: Skeletal X-ray findings and bone histology in patients on hemodialysis. Kidney Int 13:316-323, 1978.
5. Sy WM, Mittal AK: Bone scan in chronic dialysis patients with evidence of secondary hyperparathyroidism and renal osteodystrophy. Br J Radiol 48:878-884, 1975.
6. Rosenthall L, Kaye M: Technetium-99m-pyrophosphate kinetics and imaging in metabolic bone disease. J Nucl Med 16:33-39, 1975.
7. Ølgaard K, Heerfordt J, Madsen S: Scintigraphic skeletal changes in uremic patients on regular hemodialysis. Nephron 17:325-334, 1976.
8. Wiegmann T, Rosenthall L, Kaye M: Technetium-99m-pyrophosphate bone scans in hyperparathyroidism. J Nucl Med 18:231-235, 1977.
9. De Graaf P, Schicht IM, Pauwels EKJ, te Velde J, de Graeff J: Bone scintigraphy in renal osteodystrophy. J Nucl Med 19:1289-1296, 1978.
10. Neyer U. Mahr G, Ell PJ, Meixner M, Gloor F: Die Knochenszintigraphie in der Diagnostik der renalen Osteopathie. Dtsch Med Wschr 103:451-455, 1978.
11. Patel R, Ansari A, Miskin F, Toshiyuki Tanaka MT, Savage A: Early detection of renal osteodystrophy: a comparison of ^{99m}Tc-HEDSPA bone scintigraphy and serum bone alkaline phosphatase isoenzyme activity. Dialysis and Transplantation 8:692-698, 1978.
12. Fogelman I, Citrin DL, Turner JG, Hay ID, Bessent RG, Boyle IT: Semi-quantitative interpretation of the bone scan in metabolic bone disease. Eur J Nucl Med 4:287-289, 1979.
13. Lentle BC, Russell AS, Percy JS: Bone scintiscanning updated. Ann Int Med 84:297-303, 1976.
14. Ritz E, Clorius JH: Scintigraphy in uremic bone disease. Nephron 17:321-324, 1976.
15. Fogelman I, Bessent RG, Turner JG, Citrin DL, Boyle IT, Greig WR: The use of whole-body retention of Tc-99m-diphosphonate in the diagnosis of metabolic disease. J Nucl Med 19:270-275, 1978.
16. De Graaf P: Renal bone disease and extraskeletal calcification during dialysis and after transplantation: with special reference to the diagnostic value of bone scintigraphy. Thesis, Leiden, 1980.
17. De Graaf P, Pauwels EKJ, Schicht IM, Feitsma RIJ, de Graeff J: Scintigraphic detection of gastric calcification in dialysis patients. Diagn Imaging 48:171-176, 1979.
18. De Graaf P, Schicht IM, te Velde J, Pauwels EKJ, Kleiverda K, de Graeff J: Quantitative bone scintigraphy in the evaluation of treatment of renal osteodystrophy. Clin Nephrol, in press.

19. Subramanian G, McAfee JG, Blair RJ, Kallfelz FA, Thomas FD: Technetium-99m-methylene diphosphonate – a superior agent for skeletal imaging: comparison with other technetium complexes. J Nucl Med 16: 744-755, 1975.

20. De Graaf P, te Velde J, Pauwels EKJ, Schicht IM, Kleiverda K, de Graeff J: Increased bone radiotracer uptake in renal osteodystrophy: clinical evidence of hyperparathyroidism as the major cause. Eur J Nucl Med, in press.

21. Jones AG, Francis MD, Davis MA: Bone scanning: radionuclide reaction mechanisms. Semin Nucl Med 6:3-18, 1976.

22. Francis MD, Tofe AJ, Benedict JJ, Bevan JA: Imaging the skeletal system. In: Proceedings 2nd International Symposium on Radiopharmaceuticals, Seattle, Society of Nuclear Medicine (ed), New York, 1979, p 603-614.

23. Tilden RI, Jackson J, Enneking WF, DeLand FH, McVey JT: ^{99m}Tc-polyphosphate: histological localization in human femurs by autoradiography. J Nucl Med 14:576-578, 1973.

24. Van Langevelde A, Driessen OMJ, Pauwels EKJ, Thesingh CW: Aspects of ^{99m}Technetium binding from an Ethane-1-hydroxy-1,1-diphosphonate-^{99m}Tc complex to bone. Eur J Nucl Med 2:47-51, 1977.

25. Genant HK, Bautovich GJ, Singh M, Lathrop KA, Harper PV: Boneseeking radionuclides: an in vivo study of factors affecting skeletal uptake. Radiology 113:373-382, 1974.

26. Zimmer AM, Isitman AT, Holmes RA: Enzymatic inhibition of diphosphonate: a proposed mechanism of tissue uptake. J Nucl Med 16:352-356, 1975.

27. Rosenthall L, Kaye M: Observations on the mechanism of Tc-99m-labeled phosphate complex uptake in metabolic bone disease. Semin Nucl Med 6:59-67, 1976.

28. Charkes ND: Mechanisms of skeletal radiotracer uptake. J Nucl Med 20:794-795, 1979.

10. PAGET'S DISEASE

CEES J. L. R. VELLENGA

1. INTRODUCTION

Paget's disease is a usually asymptomatic bone disorder of unknown etiology Numerous publications have revealed detailed clinical, biochemical and pathohistological data (1–7). In 1968 effective treatment became possible (8) and renewed interest in Paget's disease was aroused.

The incidence of Paget's disease is 3% for those over 40 years of age (2); it is rarely detected in those under 30 years of age. The incidence increases with age, from 1% in the fifth decade to 10% in the ninth decade (4–5). Sometimes patients in the 20–30 year-old age group have been aware of symptoms related to Paget's disease, although the disease itself is not detected until a decade later (6). There is a slight predilection for males over females in a ratio of 3:2 (5).

Pauwels EKJ, Schütte HE, Taconis WK, eds, Bone scintigraphy, p 127–158.

1.1. *Symptoms and complications*

One should remember that the majority of the cases of Paget's disease are discovered accidentally and many of these patients do not have complaints (3, 7).

The most frequent complaint is pain, frequently in the joint adjacent to the affected skeletal part and caused either by Pagetic arthritis or by the altered burden on the joint due to bone deformity. In rare cases tenderness of the affected bone itself is reported. However, in this age group concomitant osteoarthritis is often present, producing arthralgia. Moreover the combination of Paget's disease and rheumatic disorders has been described (9). Other symptoms are fatigue and headaches.

The most frequent complication, apart from bowing of the bone, is probably the occurrence of fractures, although the reported incidence varies from 1% (4) to 31% (10). According to most series a fracture will probably develop in about 15% (3, 5–7) of a hospitalized population with Paget's disease. However, this figure will be much lower if we include subjects with subclinical involvement, both inside and outside hospitals (4). Moreover other authors even consider a fracture to be a fairly rare event in Paget's disease (11, 12). Healing is usually normal, although callus is often abundant. Other complications are increased cardiac output, nerve compression at the base of the skull or the vertebral foramina, and deafness.

The most dreaded complication is Paget's sarcoma, usually osteogenic, sometimes. chondrosarcoma. Although in the early literature – when a fraction of the cases of Paget's disease was detected – high percentages of incidence were recorded, later studies showed that probably not even 1% (13) of the patients with Paget's disease undergo malignant degeneration. However, when osteogenic sarcoma occurs in the elderly, Paget's disease is often the predisposing factor (14).

1.2. *Morphology and radiology*

The basic pathophysiological process in Paget's disease is a disturbance of the balance between bone resorption and bone repair, both of which occur in healthy bone. The disease probably starts with an increase in bone resorption by giant osteoclasts with numerous nuclei (2) followed by an invasion of osteoblasts depositing fibrous bone in an attempt to keep pace with the rapid destruction of bone. Microscopically the residue of the bone resorption can be seen as cement lines surrounded by newly deposited bone, which can result in the mosaic pattern characteristic for Paget's disease (2, 11). The Pagetic bone is highly vascular.

Macroscopically the involved part of the bone is enlarged and deformed. The trabeculae in the spongiosa are thickened and coarse and are often separated by wide marrow spaces. The cortex can be dense and thickened, but it is not uncommon for it to be permeated with lamellar or cyst-like spaces filled with fatty marrow and blurring the endosteal margin of the cortex. All of these macroscopic changes can readily be recognized on the roentgenogram. The diversity of the roentgenological pattern is great but most authors distinguish three categories (3, 15–18): osteolytic or osteoporotic phase. 2) mixed or combined phase. 3) sclerotic or osteoplastic phase.

Seaman (17) and Brailsford (15, 16) describe the evolution of osteolytic lesions in the long bones – and especially the early, expansive lytic lesion called acute halisteresis – into mixed and subsequently sclerotic lesions thereby concluding that the osteolytic phase is the early onset of Paget's disease. Schmorl (2) confirmed that Paget's disease starts with osteolysis by demonstrating microscopically high osteoclastic activity and bone resorption in an area distal to the grossly involved bone.

Frequently the osteolytic lesion extends with a V-shaped front into the normal bone; this configuration, if present, is pathognomonic for Paget's disease. The cranial equivalent of the lytic phase is osteoporosis circumscripta of the skull; this form has also developed into the later phases of Paget's disease in several patients (7, 19). In the skull the sclerotic phase often presents as multiple opacities with fuzzy margins in a matrix of thickened and deformed bone.

The three phases of Paget's disease may be encountered in every part of the skeleton; generally more than one phase is present in the same patient and even in the same bone.

1.3. *Biochemistry*

The excessive bone formation and hyperactivity of osteoblasts results in very high levels of serum alkaline phosphatase, which may be elevated to twenty times the normal value (20). The high bone turnover and resorption of the collagen matrix of bone cause high levels of urine hydroxyproline. Both biochemical values show a signifiant correlation with the percentage of skeletal involvement (5, 7, 21), although they are also influenced by the degree of activity of the disease (5, 12). The serum calcium and phosphorous levels remain within the normal range (5, 20). The bone turnover of Ca as well as the size of both the short-term and long-term pools is considerably increased (20).

2. BONE SCINTIGRAPHY

2.1. *Introduction*

The first reports of bone scanning in Paget's disease pertained to ^{85}Sr and appeared 20 years ago (22, 23). Occasionally ^{87m}Sr was used (24). ^{47}Ca is not suitable for imaging because of its high energy but is currently used for measuring the rate of bone turnover and the size of the bone pools (5, 20, 25). Later larger series of patients were scanned using ^{18}F (12, 24, 26, 27) and ^{99m}Tc compounds (12, 26–29).

2.2. *Methods*

Imaging is usually performed 1 to 4 hr after the intravenous administration of 2 to 5 mCi of ^{18}F using a scanner, e.g. a dual probe 5–in scanner (12), or 3 to 5 hr. after injection of 10 to 20 mCi of ^{99m}Tc EHDP, ^{99m}Tc MDP or ^{99m}Tc pyrophosphate using a rectilinear scanner (30) or a large-field gamma camera. Data control may be useful especially in combination with a gamma camera (28, 29, 31, 32), but is not obligatory. In general the Pagetic lesions are readily visualized without data control but evaluation of the activity of the disease is more difficult (26), especially in severe cases (29). If digital data processing is not possible, a careful estimation of the rate of uptake is quite satisfactory, as we could conclude from a comparison between a qualitative scoring method and a computer-assisted quantitative evaluation (33–35).

The qualitative scoring system was set up as follows:

score 6: very high uptake in Pagetoid bone; the surrounding normal bone is not visualized dut to the high count rate and short exposure time.

score 5: very high uptake in Pagetoid bone, but some activity is seen in normal bone.

score 4: moderately high uptake in the pathological area; normal bone is clearly visualized.

score 3: the uptake in Pagetoid bone is only slightly elevated, but it is still distinctly demarcated from normal bone.

score 2: the Pagetoid bone can hardly be differentiated from normal bone; normalization is almost reached.

score 1: normal.

In some studies quantitation of radionuclide uptake was performed by means of external counting with a 2-inch crystal probe over pre-selected areas (27). Sometimes dynamic studies of bone vascularity have also been obtained (28, 36); other investigators have made bone marrow scans using ^{99m}Tc-colloid (28, 37).

2.3. Mechanism of uptake in Pagetoid bone

The ^{99m}Tc-Sn-phosphorous compounds probably accumulate by chemi-resorption on the surface of the hydroxy-apatite crystal (38). Factors influencing the uptake are vascularity (38–40), bone turnover (38–40), the exchangeable bone pool (38, 39) and extracellular fluid in bone (41), while some authors attribute great importance to the amount of osteoid (42) and others stress the local concentration of enzymes such as alkaline phosphatase (43).

In Paget's disease virtually all of these factors are greatly elevated: the bone is highly vascularized (44, 45), and the pronounced bone turn-over is the hallmark of the disease; it is known from radiocalcium studies that the exchangeable bone pool is increased (5, 20, 46), the amount of osteoid is excessive and the local production of alkaline phosphatase is marked. Therefore it is to be expected that the uptake of ^{99m}Tc-Sn-EHDP in Pagetoid bone will be very high.

Although the mechanism of uptake of ^{18}F is different, the resultant image is essentially the same. Generally the ratio of uptake for pathological to normal bone is higher for ^{18}F than for ^{99m}Tc-Sn-EHDP; however, anatomical detail is less clearly visualized because of the high energy of the gamma-emission of [18]F.

[18]F is thought to be incorporated into bone by replacement of the hydroxyl groups in the hydroxy-apatite crystal. The avidity of ^{18}F for bone is very great, all of the carrier-free ^{18}F being extracted from the blood in the first transit (47). Some of the factors governing the uptake of ^{18}F in bone are the same as those for the ^{99m}Tc-compounds, because according to Blau et al. (48) a high uptake of ^{18}F results from an increased bone crystal surface and local blood flow.

Charkes (41, 49, 50) demonstrated that for both ^{18}F and ^{99m}Tc-Sn-MDP the flow is "diffusion-limited" due to a buffer function of the extracellular fluid in bone, which means that a further increase in blood flow has hardly any effect on the uptake of the radiopharmaceutics. In contrast, an increase in the number of capillaries, as in Paget's disease (44, 45), causes marked elevation of the uptake of bone-scanning agents (49, 50).

132

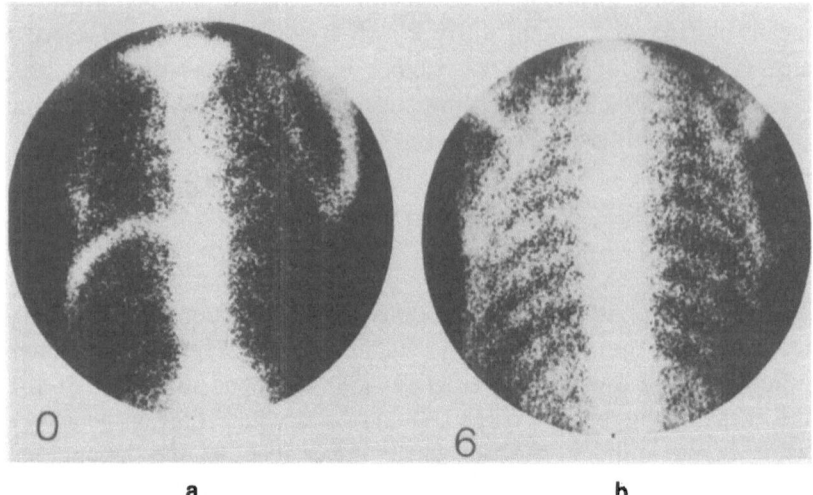

a   b

Figure 1a. Paget's disease of the right scapula, left 8th rib, first dorsal vertebra and first lumbar vertebra. Anatomical details are fairly visualized. Radiographs of the scapula showed no abnormality, probably due to subtlety of the bone resorption and/or to lack of accessibility of radiological examination; the dorsal vertebra showed slight osteolysis, the rib was slightly sclerotic on the x-rays.
b. After 6 months of combined treatment complete normalization of these bones is seen.

2.4. *Scintigraphic appearance*

Although bone scintigraphy is an aspecific method of investigation, the scintigraphic findings in Paget's disease are often unequivocal and conclusive (32). The characteristic appearance is a highly elevated uptake of the radiopharmaceutic which is evenly distributed throughout the affected part of the bone; the latter is often expanded and deformed. As a rule the affected area is well defined and anatomical detail is clearly visualized (Figures 1, 2, 3a). The uptake in pathological bone can be 5–20 times that in normal bone.

In long bones the lesion begins at one or both ends, extending from the joint toward the diaphysis; sometimes the V-front can be recognized (Figures 2, 3a). In the pelvis a hemipelvic distribution is common, whereas in the spine only one or several vertebrae are effected. In the skull several scintigraphic patterns are possible: one hot spot (Figure 15), one or multiple irregular areas and sometimes the entire skull shows very high activity with gross deformity and thickening of the skullcap (Figure 14).

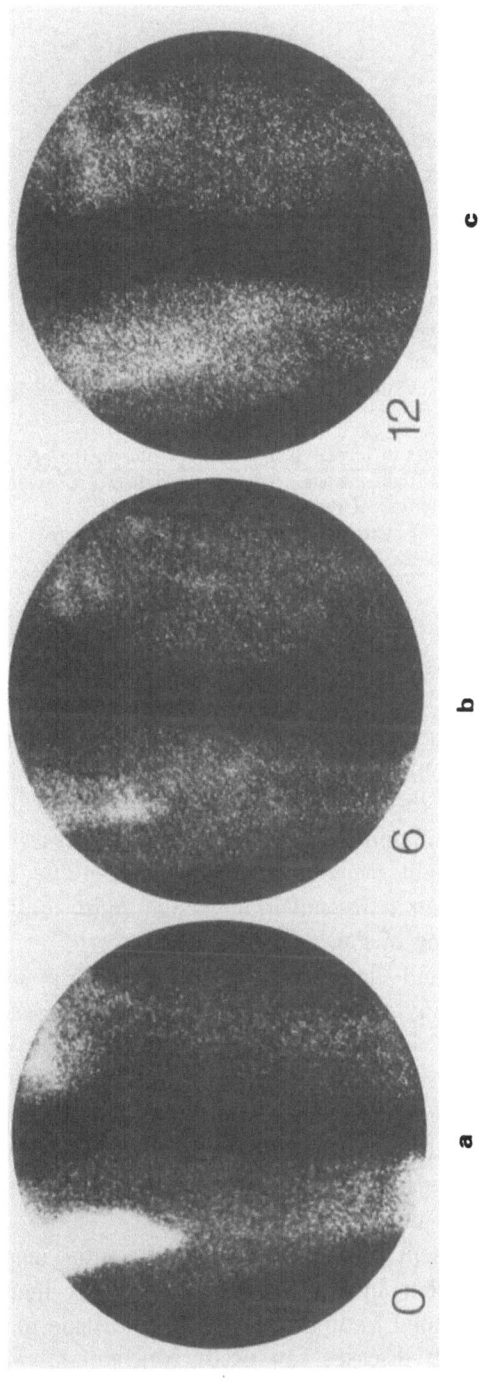

Figure 2a. The sharp V-formed demarcation of the lesion, a characteristic finding in Paget's disease, is apparent on the scintigram before treatment starts. Anatomical detail is well visualized.
b. After 6 months of diphosphonate-treatment impressive amelioration has taken place. Computer-assisted quantitation showed a fall of uptake from 5.2 times normal to 1.5 times normal.
c. After 12 months the proximal right tibia is virtually normal.

134

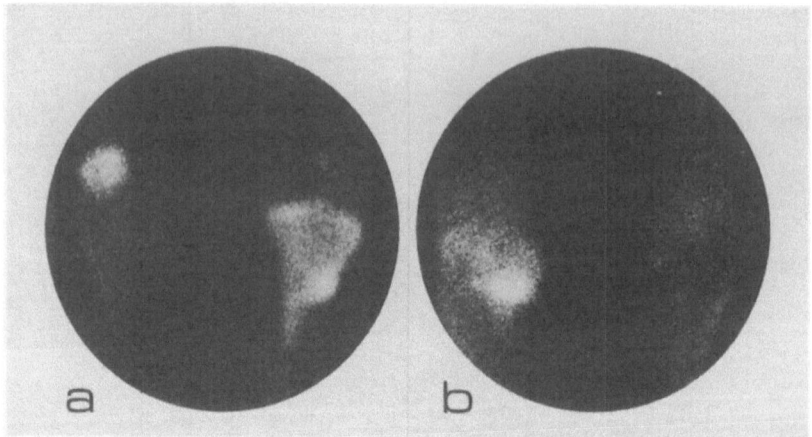

Figure 3a. Sharply circumscript areas of increased uptake are visible in the proximal left tibia (with V-formed front) and right patella. Anatomical details are evident. The scintigraphic appearance is characteristic of Paget's disease.
b. In another patient a fuzzy spot of increased uptake is seen in the right proximal tibia, characteristic for degenerative disease. This was confirmed radiologically.

2.5. Differential diagnosis

The full-blown scintigraphic picture of polyostotic Paget's disease seldom presents diagnostic problems, but doubt can arise when the disease is confined to the spine or the skull or is monostotic.

Fibrous dysplasia can be differentiated because of the diaphyseal rather than metaphyseal involvement. irregular uptake of radioactivity, disruption of the anatomic configurations and irregular deformity, unlike the diffuse widening and bowing of Pagetic bones.

In *osteomyelitis* a diffuse and slight elevation of the uptake in adjacent bone and soft tissue is usually apparent due to the increased vascularity which, in Paget's disease, is restricted to the affected part of the bone.

In *arthritis* and *osteoarthritis* both bones on either side of the joint show diffuse and ill-defined uptake as opposed to the clear delineation of the bones in Pagetic lesions (Figure 3). These articular disorders often occur together with Paget's disease.

Metastatic neoplasms present the most difficult differential diagnosis. Both disease processes occur in similar age groups and frequently Paget's disease is an accidental finding on a bone scan made to detect malignancy. Moreover both diseases can occur concomitantly in the same patient.

Although both diseases have an affinity for the axial skeleton, metastatic disease generally presents as spotty lesions randomly distributed throughout the skeleton, involving any portion of a bone with normal intervening bone. There is no bony deformation or overgrowth and the anatomical details are locally blurred; in contrast Paget's disease may show enlargement and bowing of the affected bone and always produces enhanced visibility of the anatomical structures.

Differentiation of treated Paget's disease can be difficult, because a recurrence of Paget's disease can become manifest as foci of increased activity (Figure 14).

Paget's sarcoma is the most troublesome diagnosis in these cases. It may present as either a cold or a hot lesion but must be suspected if localized intense activity is seen beyond the usual confines of the affected bone, although the same appearance can be caused by a fracture. Radiologically too the diagnosis of sarcoma is difficult due to the seriously altered bone architecture; often its presence is heralded by the detection of metastases.

The demonstration of sarcomatous degeneration with ^{67}Ga-citrate may not be considered conclusive, because this tracer concentrates in Pagetoid bone in excessive amounts even in the absence of malignant change (28). Sometimes development of sarcoma is revealed by a rise in the alkaline phosphatase level (5, 13).

2.6. *Anatomical distribution*

There is some disagreement among various authors (2, 3, 6, 7) on the anatomical distribution of Paget's disease, which can be attributed to the differences in classification of the sites, selection of patients and – most important – methods of investigation. Some studies were based on complete or incomplete roentgenographic surveys (3, 6, 17), others on autopsy reports (2), and very few on scintigraphy (12, 35, 51). However, it is evident that the axial skeleton is affected most often: i.e. in order of decreasing frequency the pelvis, sacrum, lumbar spine and skull. Of the appendicular skeleton the femur and tibia are affected most often (Table 1).

There seem to be slight differences in average uptake at different anatomical sites, suggesting that some parts of the skeleton are more severely involved than others. The skull tends to show the highest uptake, whereas the tibia, femur, humerus and pelvis often have higher count rates than the spine (33–35). Other parts of the skeleton show less severe changes when affected. Monostotic disease is not common,

Table 1. Anatomical distribution of Paget's disease, given by several authors, using different methods of investigation. Percentages are not known for every anatomical part; figures, marked with*, are approximations, because these incidences were given separately for left and right side, or for lumbar and dorsal spine and so on.

Author: Method of investigation: Number of patients:	Schmorl autopsy 138	Dickson radiography 367	Rosenkrantz radiography 111	Shirazi scintigraphy 136	Vellenga scintigraphy 76
Sacrum	56%	21%*		28%	24%
Spine	50%	42%*	40%*	63%	43%
Femur	40%*	47%	45%*	48%	39%
Cranium	28%	42%	36%	48%	41%
Pelvis	21%	66%	62%	78%	72%
Tibia	8%	35%	17%	22%	33%
Sternum	23%			4%	8%
Clavicle	13%	9%	7%	3%	
Scapula		2%	7%	37%	20%
Humerus	4%	5%	15%	17%	18%
Ribs	7%	3%	3%	5%	13%

10% of the cases according to Shirazi (12) and Collins (4) and 14% in our material (51).

2.7. *Correlation with radiography and symptomatology*

Grainger and Laws (52) found that osteolytic lesions on the radiograph were usually accompanied by complaints of pain, whereas sclerotic lesions were often asymptomatic.

Sclerotic lesions are also associated with lower levels of alkaline phosphatase than combined or lytic lesions (3, 12), suggesting that sclerotic lesions are burnt out and quiescent end-stages.

Khairi et al. (21, 53) stated that some Pagetic lesions were detected only roentgenographically but not scintigraphically and that these lesions were usually asymptomatic and sclerotic. Other lesions were detected only on the scintigram, and these were symptomatic. They concluded that the bone scan was sensitive specifically for evaluation of clinically and metabolically active lesions.

Shirazi (12) obtained strikingly positive bone scans of symptomatic lesions but could not confirm that these lesions were more active than asymptomatic or sclerotic lesions. Only rarely was a (sclerotic) lesion not visualized on the bone scan.

Lavender (30) also noted a disparity between radiographic and scintigraphic findings but does not comment on the type of lesion.

The bone scintiscan disclosed 34% more lesions than conventional radiographs in the series of Lentle et al. (28).

In our material there seemed to be no evidence that lytic lesions are scintigraphically more active than sclerotic lesions. There was some tendency for lesions with gross involvement and deformity on the radiograph to show higher scintigraphic activity, whereas lesions which were not visible on the radiograph in general had only a moderately elevated uptake of radioactivity. In 25 out of 43 patients we demonstrated disagreement of radiographic and scintigraphic detection of Paget's disease, occurring in 38 lesions. Table 2 shows the localizations of lesions, which were demonstrated only by scintigraphy and not by radiography. Since the total number of lesions in these 43 patients was 173, it appeared that 22% of the Pagetic sites was visible only on the scintigram.

There are probably two reasons for the discrepancy between the two methods. In the first place, some bones, e.g. the scapula, sternum and ribs, are not easily accessible for radiological examination (Figures 1 and 4). The second reason is that osteolysis in early Paget's disease can be

Table 2. Tabulation of regions of Paget's disease, visible only scintigraphically and not radiologically. These regions of disagreement were present in 25 out of 43 patients. These 43 patients appeared to have 173 Pagetic lesions altogether.

Anatomical site	Number of lesions
Scapula	6
Lumbar spine	4
Thoracic spine	4
Cervical spine	2
Skull	4
Tibia	4
Pelvis	4
Sacrum	3
Foot	3
Sternum	2
Humerus	1
Ribs	1
Total	38

too subtle to be detected on the roentgenogram, since approximately 30% of the bone must be resorbed to effectuate roentgenographic alterations.

We demonstrated 4 lesions only on the X-ray and not on the scintigram; two were sclerotic and two were of the mixed type. However, in our patients radiography was not routinely performed of the whole skeleton and therefore the number of positive radiographs and negative scintigrams will possibly be greater.

3. TREATED PAGET'S DISEASE

3.1. *Introduction*

Because the etiology of Paget's disease was obscure, it took many years before effective treatment became possible. The first drug shown to be effective was calcitonin (8), and subsequently large series of patients were treated with either salmon, porcine or human calcitonin (29, 30, 54, 55). The drawback of calcitonin is incomplete normalization of the biochemical levels, which fall to values equivalent to 50% of the original values and – in virtually all instances – rebound during or after treatment. Ethane-hydroxy-diphosphonate (EHDP) appeared to be

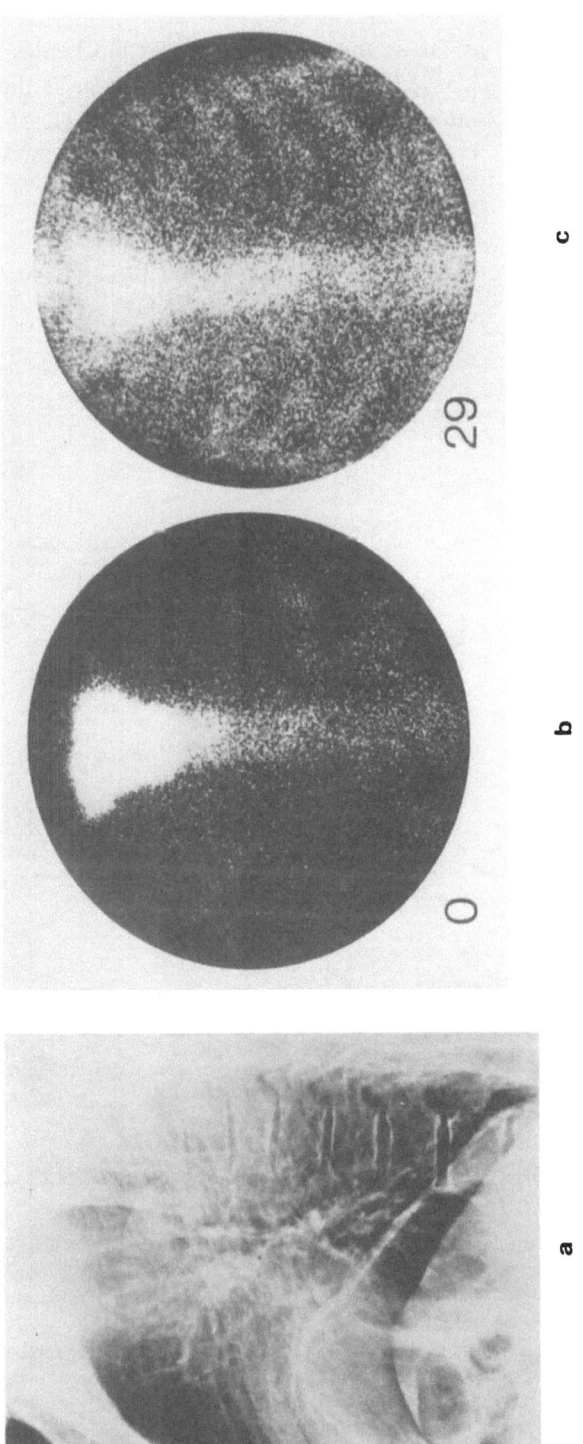

Figure 4a. Paget's disease in the corpus of the 8th thoracic vertebra. If one looks carefully at the lateral X-ray of the thorax of this patient, one sees an undeniable thickening and slight increase in density of the cortex in the manubrium sterni. This could easily be overlooked, and demonstrates that bones like the sternum are not easily accessible for radiological examination.
b. On the scintigram an eye-catching increase of uptake is seen in the manubrium sterni (score 5).
c. After combination therapy with calcitonin and EHDP complete normalization is reached.

an even more potent drug as far as the reduction of the biochemical
levels is concerned (24, 26, 53, 56, 57), but its major disadvantage is the
condiderable increase in the amount of unmineralized osteoid (27, 56,
58). The adverse effects of both agents, however, can be suppressed,

a **b** **c**

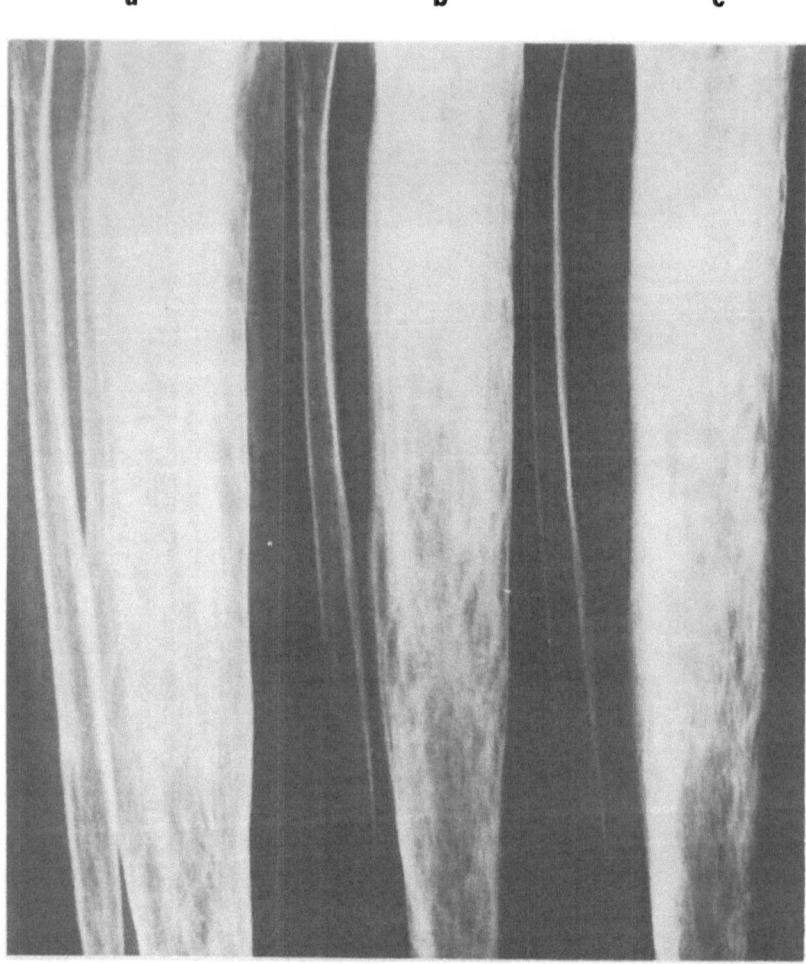

Figure 5a. Before treatment the characteristic radiological appearance of Paget's disease
with broadening of the bone, osteolytic spaces interspersed with more sclerotic bone,
thickening and demineralization of the cortex, blurring of the endosteal border and
coarsening of the trabeculation, is apparent.
b. After 6 months of combined treatment there is the semblance of a cortex with a more
clearly defined endosteal surface; the osteolytic spaces have become filled with wellminer-
alized bone; the cortical thickness decreases and remineralization takes place.
c. One and a half year later further improvement has taken place; the Pagetic bone has
assumed a normal trabecular structure, the cortex is more clearly defined with an increase
in mineralization. The entire bone has assumed again a normal shape.

while their benefits are retained by administration of a combination of low doses of calcitonin and EHDP (20). The third drug which appeared to be effective is mithramycine (28, 36, 59), but its cytotoxic effect is a limitation.

The advent of therapeutic possibilities necessitated precise evaluation of the activity of the disease. Evaluation of symptomatology is difficult (24, 58), whereas the levels of serum alkaline phosphatase and urine hydroxyproline are reliable and useful parameters (5, 20). However, these values reflect an average level in the entire body and provide only indirect information about local activity of the disease in different lesions. The same is true for ^{47}Ca-kinetics. Bone biopsies provide information about only one site in the skeleton. Therefore radiography and bone scintigraphy remain as the only methods which reveal the status at specific sites in the skeleton.

Radiographic changes occur during treatment of Paget's disease (35, 46, 54, 60) (Figure 5) and – with meticulous positioning and a precise radiographic technique – these changes are usually evident and may be useful for evaluation of the treatment (60, 61). However, the method is time-consuming and the changes are slow and subtle.

3.2. Bone scintigraphy as a parameter during treatment

Bone scintigraphy was used as a parameter of the activity of Paget's disease by several research groups (24, 26–28, 33–35, 53, 58), and most of them agree that there is a considerable reduction of activity during successful treatment, and that scintigraphy can provide useful information.

Although some groups utilized ^{18}F (26, 27), many could not obtain fluorine and had to use ^{99m}Tc-agents. Especially when EHDP is given therapeutically, one should pose the question of whether there is an interaction between these drugs. There are three reasons for believing that this interaction is probably not of major importance: 1) Van Langevelde et al. (62) demonstrated in animal experiments that doses such as used in the treatment of Paget's disease do not influence the uptake of ^{99m}Tc-Sn-EHDP when administered for 7 days; 2) The count rate in normal bones does not alter during treatment (27, 35); 3) scans with ^{18}F and ^{99m}Tc-Sn-EHDP, as well as ^{87m}Sr and ^{99m}Tc-Sn-EHDP (63), are identical during treatment with EHDP (27, 31).

3.3. Scintigraphic changes during treatment

There seems to be a dose-related scintigraphic response during treatment with calcitonin when the scan is evaluated with a quantitative technique (26, 29); during calcitonin therapy scintigraphic amelioration is maximal during the first three months but continues for up to 12 months (30). During treatment with mithramycine significant scintigraphic changes were also noticed (12, 36), with a decrease in the involved normal bone ratio from 9 to 4. However, with this treatment there seem to be no distinct changes during the first two months (12).

Treatment with EHDP resulted in a dose-related reduction of the uptake of both ^{18}F and ^{87m}Sr (24, 27) and several investigators reported improvement of the scintigram in most cases during treatment of EHDP (27, 58), with approximately a 50% drop in uptake during the first 6 months (26). Goldman (26) reported 4 patients on high doses of EHDP, who had no interval change in the 6-month scan, although quantitative evaluation showed a decrease of radionuclide uptake of at least 57%. This illustrates the hazard of qualitative bone scintigraphy.

When low doses of EHDP are given in combination with calcitonin (20), scintigraphic improvement is always seen during the first year, the greatest changes occurring during the first 6 months (33–35) (Figures 1, 6, 7, 9); during this period 75% of the total decrease in scintigraphic score was attained.

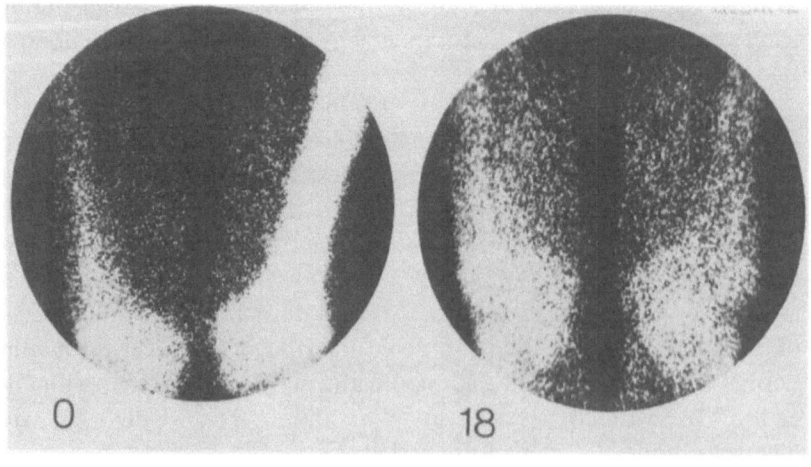

a   b

Figure 6a. The initial scintigram shows very high uptake in the left femur (score 5).
b. After 18 months of combined treatment, the scintigram is completely normal (score 1).

3.4. *Local changes*

According to Lavender (30) all lesions change in a similar way during treatment with calcitonin. We observed this same trend during combined treatment (33–35). There was a parallel drop in activity in all affected bones which means that seriously affected parts of the skeleton retained a higher activity than mildly affected bones (Figures 7 and 8); it was not uncommon for the latter to normalize (Figures 1, 2, 4, 6, 8).

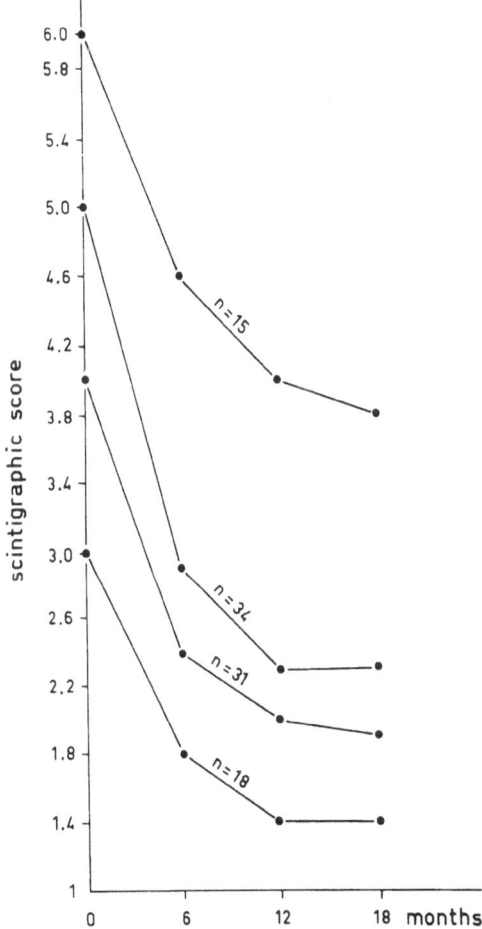

Figure 7. The average of the scintigraphic scores during treatment of bones with a pre-treatment score of 6, 5, 4 and 3, respectively. Above each curve the number of bones included is indicated. The curves are roughly parallel and bones with a higher initial score remain more active than bones with a lower initial score. Normalization is not unusual in mildly affected regions.

144

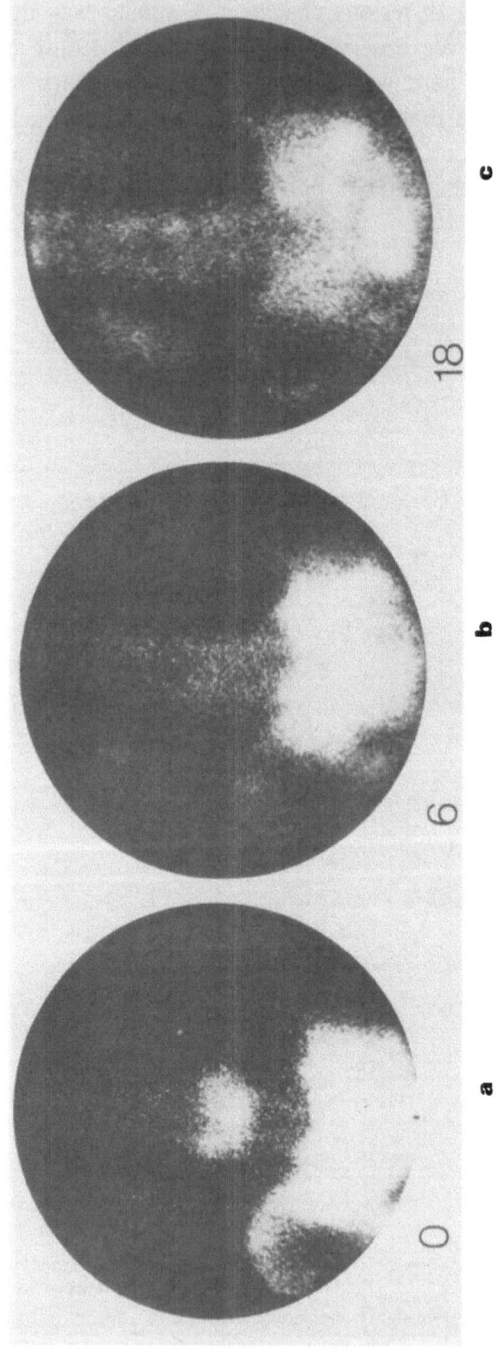

Figure 8a. Paget's disease was found in the 4th lumbar vertebra (score 4), and the sacrum (score 5).
b. After 6 months of treatment the vertebra is completely normal, whereas the sacrum, which was involved more seriously, reaches score 4.
c. One year later the sacrum shows a further improvement, with almost normalization of the left wing, but still activity on the right.
This illustrates the general principle of the parallel fall of scintigraphic activity during treatment: the higher the initial score, the higher the residual activity; mildly affected parts readily normalize.

Sometimes differences of uptake within the same bone exist, which show a parallel fall of activity, resulting in normalization of one part of the bone whereas another more seriously affected part remains abnormal (Figure 8).

After one year of treatment a more or less steady state is achieved, in which the activity of the individual lesions depends on the initial degree of involvement (Figures 7, 8).

This is not in agreement with the findings of Waxman et al. (29), who noted that there is less improvement in seriously involved bones than in moderately affected regions.

3.5 *Correlation with other parameters*

There is a rather good correlation between scintigraphic and biochemical improvement (12, 24, 26, 32), although discrepancies are encountered (30, 53). Scintigraphic changes are not apparent during the first 2 months of treatment with mithramycine; the biochemical parameters are far more useful for recording amelioration during this period (12), probably due to the remodeling and healing process during early treatment.

In contrast Lavender (30) described the greatest scintigraphic improvement during the first three months of calcitonin therapy.

The tendency for patients on combined treatment to improve, reach a plateau or suffer a recurrence, is independent of the parameters used to evaluate the disease (Figure 9). Figures 9a to c indicate the fair agreement between scintigraphic and biochemical findings in respect of the type of reaction on treatment. In the patients with total biochemical remission the average decrease in the scintigraphic score was 75% (Figure 9a), whereas this decrease was only 40% for patients reaching a plateau of biochemical values (35) (Figure 9b). The average decrease in the scintigraphic score was 52% in patients suffering recurrence of Paget's disease, whereas the scintigraphic curves also show the rise of the score during recurrence (Figure 9c).

There are however differences between these two parameters. Whereas during combined treatment an exponential reduction of the biochemical values with a half-time of $1\frac{1}{2}$ months is seen (20), the scintigraphic improvement is much slower (Figures 7, 9). Moreover biochemical normalization is much more common than scintigraphic normalization.

Waxman (29) describes the scintigraphic changes as being distinctly inferior to the biochemical improvement. especially in severe disease.

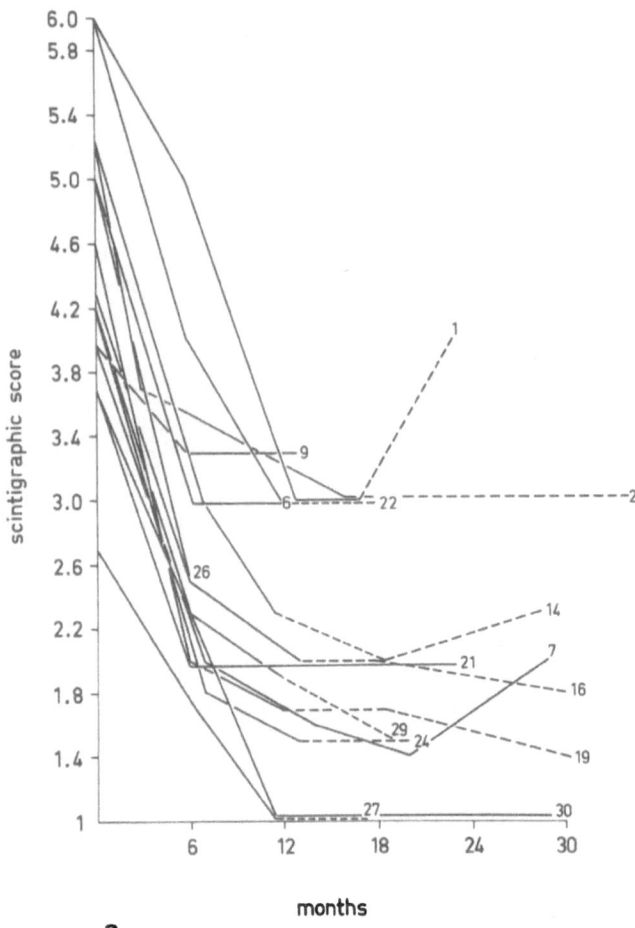

Figure 9. The average scintigraphic score for the affected bones in each individual patient is given on the vertical axis; the time in months after start of treatment on the horizontal axis. Dashed lines indicate that treatment was discontinued.

Figure 9a. The average scintigraphic scores for the affected bones in 15 patients with lasting remission (group I). There is a rapid decrease in scintigraphic activity during the first year of treatment, followed by stabilization. In three patients a rise in scintigraphic activity has been seen recently, which has not (yet) been reflected by a clinical deterioration.

There is an even closer similarity between the changes in bone scintigraphy and in the exchangeable bone pool (20, 35) (Figure 10), possibly because the exchangeable pool is one of the factors determining the uptake of ^{99m}Tc-SN-EHDP.

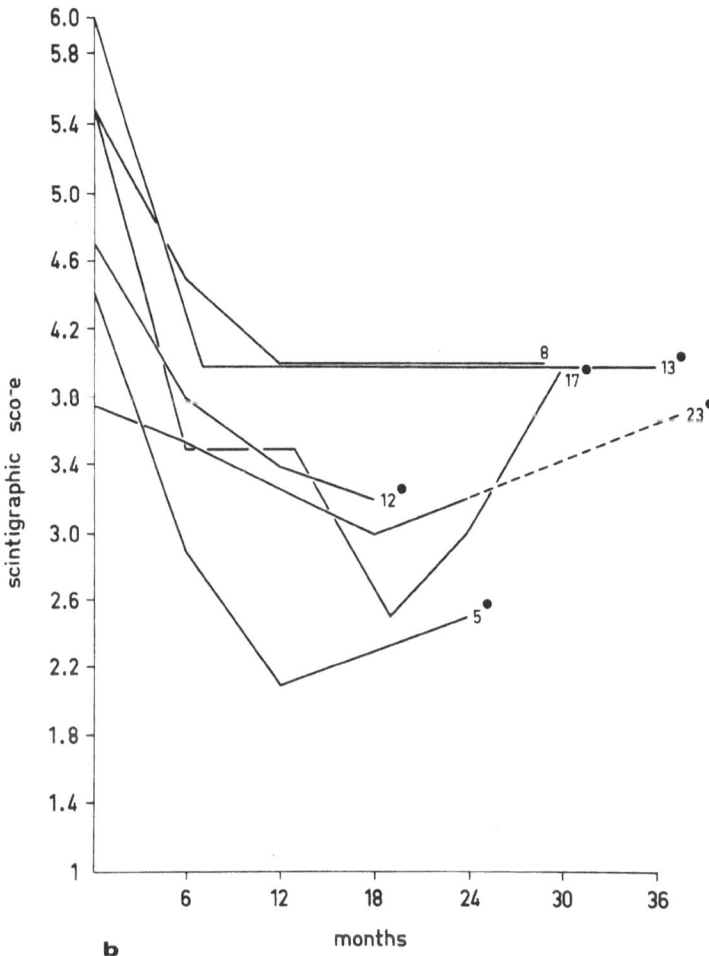

Figure 9b. The average scintigraphic scores for the affected bones in 6 patients with a plateau phenomenon (group II). The scintigraphic activity decreases somewhat more slowly. In 5 patients (marked with ●) a clinical relapse was encountered. Only patient 13 showed no scintigraphic deterioration; in patient 12 the average score continued to decrease but one bone showed reactivation.

3.6. *Remission and normalization*

Irrespective of the kind of treatment there are patients who normalize and others who do not. For the group receiving calcitonin, the success of treatment is predictable, because it depends more or less on the pre-treatment levels of alkaline phosphatase. For patients receiving EHDP the course of the disease is more difficult to predict; the same is true for those on combined treatment, although the results are fairly

148

good (20). The initial biochemical values do not forcecast the chance of clinical normalization, neither does the initial anatomical distribution nor the scintigraphic severity of the disease (20, 35). In the case of severe scintigraphic involvement one can predict that the scintigram will remain pathological, but this does not at all preclude biochemical and clinical normalization. As a matter of fact during combined treatment lasting remission was achieved in approximately 50% of our patients, whereas completely normal scintigrams were seldom seen. In fact 30%

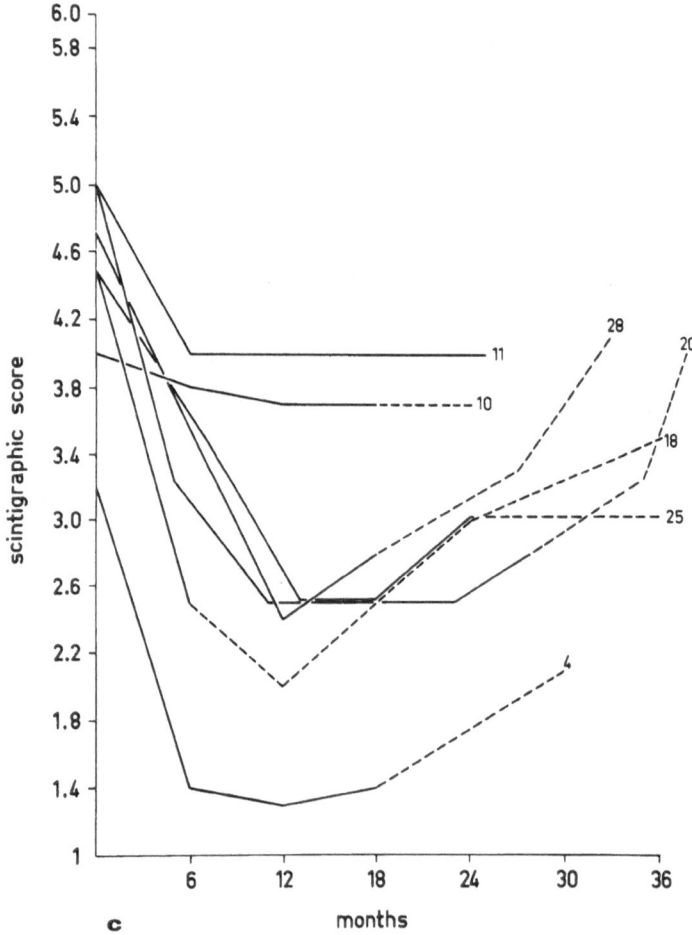

Figure 9c. The average scintigraphic scores for the affected bones in 7 patients with a relapse of Paget's disease after initial improvement (group III). The scintigraphic deterioration is evident in most patients; patient 11 has not been examined scintigraphically since deterioration. In patient 10 one bone deteriorated but the average score dit not rise.

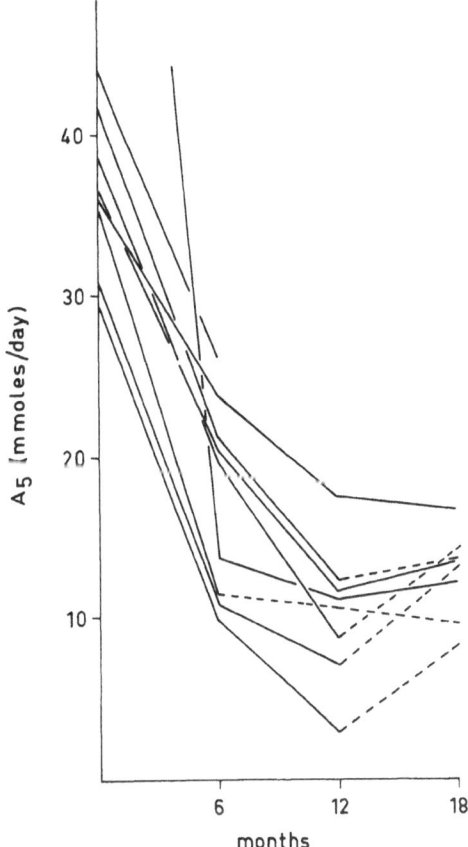

Figure 10. The rate of uptake of ^{47}Ca into bone, in pools with a turnover time exceeding 5 days (A5) in 8 patients before treatment and at 6-month intervals after the start of combined treatment. Kinetic analysis was carried out according to Marshall (20, 25).

of the lesions disappeared from the scintigram, although the gross radiological abnormalities persisted (35). The lesions with the highest pre-treatment activity, in contrast, remained visible on the scintigram. This residual scintigraphic activity during biochemical remission probably reflects the permanent changes in the micro- and macroarchitecture of the bone, as demonstrated by histology and radiology. This situation can be likened to the charred and deserted battlefield after a battle, whereby the active osteoclasts and osteoblasts are the soldiers.

Thus it must be stressed that scintigraphic and biochemical normalization are quite different matters, and that scintigraphic normalization is not required for the patient to be in remission of Paget's disease.

4. RECURRENCE OF TREATED PAGET'S DISEASE

Calcitonin therapy is followed as a rule by recurrence of the disease whereas prolonged remission is possible after both mithramycine and diphosphonate treatment, – also after discontinuation of therapy. However, the hazard of a recurrence of Paget's disease is present with every kind of treatment. The reactivation of the disease is apparent on the scintigram (35, 63).

In most cases the recurrence is visible on the scintigram as either: 1) a diffuse increase in activity (Figure 11); 2) foci of increased uptake in the diseased bone, which appear different from the original image; sometimes the focal variety presents as an inhomogeneous increase of uptake (Figure 13), in other instances as circumscipt foci of radioactivity in the affected bone (Figure 12), and in some patients these spots can be so vivid that it is impossible to differentiate them from metastatic disease (Figure 14); or 3) progression beyond the original boundaries of the lesion (Figure 15); this is the least common form.

Despite treatment new lesions can also originate in previously normal areas. In general scintigraphic deterioration is apparent in only one or a few lesions, whereas others remain unchanged.

There is a rather good correlation between the biochemical and the scintigraphic evidence of a relapse (Table 3). In 32 out of 40 patients the findings were in agreement. A recurrence is first detected scintigraphically in one-third of the cases and biochemically in another one-third. False-positive scintigraphic evidence of a recurrence was infrequent. This means that a deteriorating scintigram is a reliable indicator of recurrence of Paget's disease, and that scintigraphy is useful for the early detection of a recurrence. However, absence of scintigraphic deterioration does not preclude a recurrence since in 30% of the cases, the scintigraphic changes occur later than the biochemical.

Table 3. Relationship between scintigraphic and biochemical evidence for a relapse of treated Paget's disease.

	Biochemical change	No biochemical change	Biochemically not sure
Scintigraphic change	17 [a]	2	2
No scintigraphic change	3	15	
Scintigraphically not sure	1		

[a] Scintigraphic deterioration preceded biochemical relapse by 4-20 months in 6 instances and the changes were almost simultaneous (<3 months) in 6 other patients: biochemical deterioration preceded scintigraphic relapse by 6 to 12 months in 5 patients.

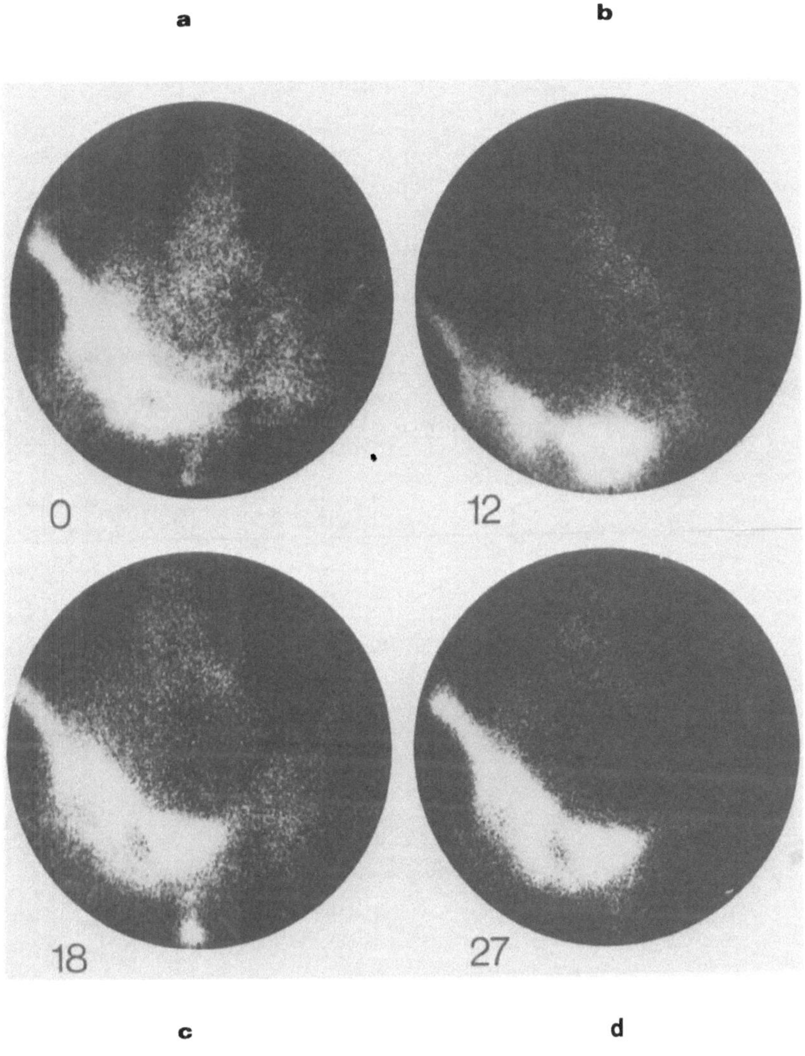

Figure 11a. The right hemi-pelvis shows Paget's disease (score 5).

b. After 12 months of combined treatment amelioration to score 3 is seen. Meanwhile the alkaline phosphatase level in the serum has fallen to normal.

c. After 18 months the serum alkaline phosphatase was still normal, and therefore therapy was discontinued. However, at this time the scintigram indicates increasing activity and thus a relapse of disease.

d. After 27 months the biochemical values rise to pathological values, confirming the relapse of Paget's disease. The scintigram has deteriorated further.

The events in this patient show the importance of scintigraphic follow-up and early scintigraphic detection of a relapse. In approximately one-third of the relapses of disease the scintigraphic evidence was noticed prior to the rise of biochemical levels; in one-third of the cases the biochemical and scintigraphic changes occurred simultaneously and in one-third of the relapses the biochemical changes preceded the scintigraphic changes.

a   b

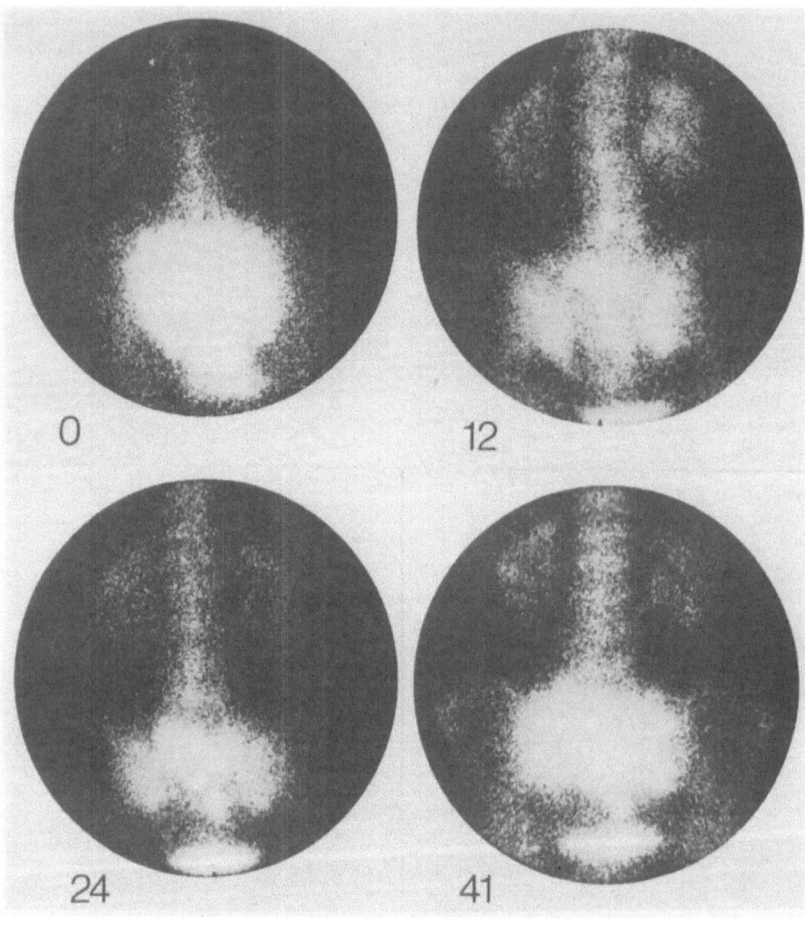

c   d

Figure 12a. Paget's disease caused very high uptake of the radionuclide in the sacrum (score 5).
b. In 12 months biochemical values had returned to normal and the scintigraphic activity was almost normal (score 2). Treatment was stopped.
c. One year later multiple foci of increased uptake are seen, indicating a relapse, although biochemical values remained normal.
d. One and a half year later the relapse was apparent clinically too, and the scintigram has deteriorated further.

An explanation for this phenomenon could either be: 1) a slight rise in local activity which is visible on the scintigram but does not yet lead to an increase in the level of total body alkaline phosphatase and hydroxyproline; or 2) the fact that we are dealing with two different

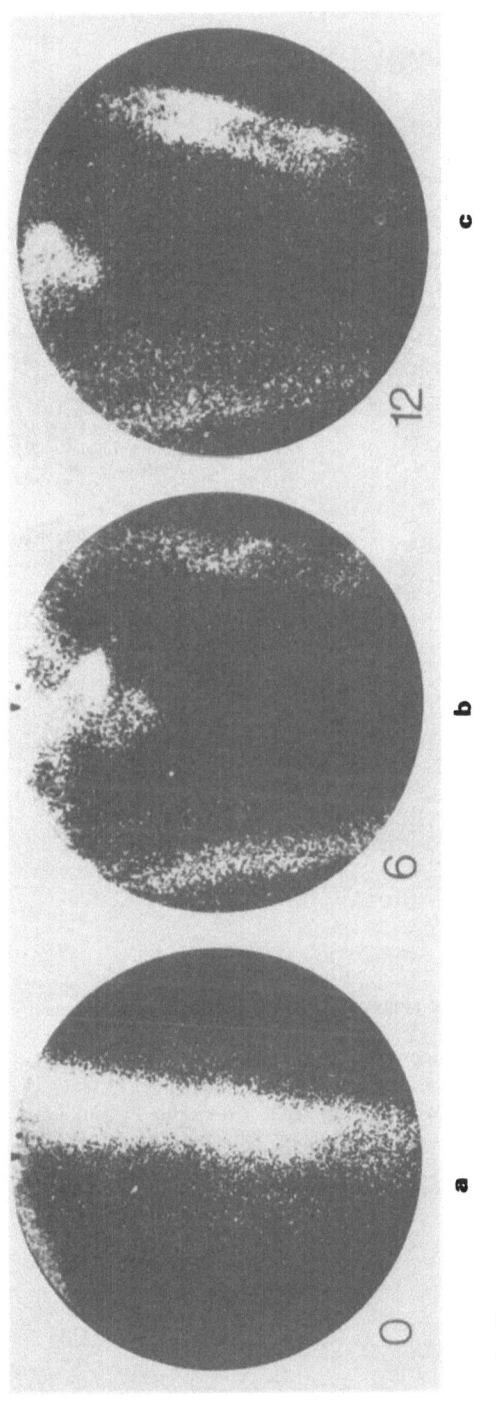

Figure 13a. The scintigram of the left femur shows Paget's disease (score 4).
b. After 6 months of combined treatment the scintigraphic activity fell to almost normal (score 2).
c. After one year a local increase of uptake is seen in the diseased area. The appearance is not as focal as in fig. 12, but not as homogeneous as in fig. 11. Simultaneously the biochemical levels rose.

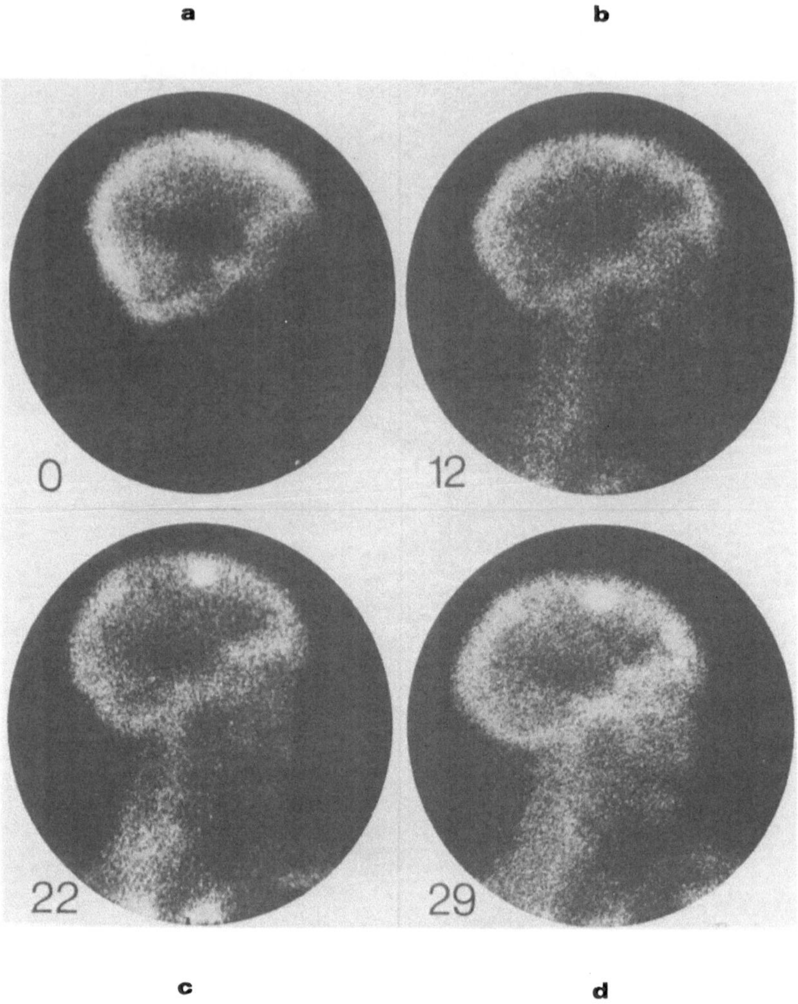

Figure 14a. Very high uptake of radioactivity in the skull causes non-visualization of the cervical spine (score 6).

b. After one year of treatment impressive amelioration has been attained (score 3). Faintly a very focal increase in the parietal bone can be observed.

c. After 22 months a hot spot arises in the vault of the skull.

d. After 29 months the spot is even more intense. Differentiation from metastatic disease is impossible.

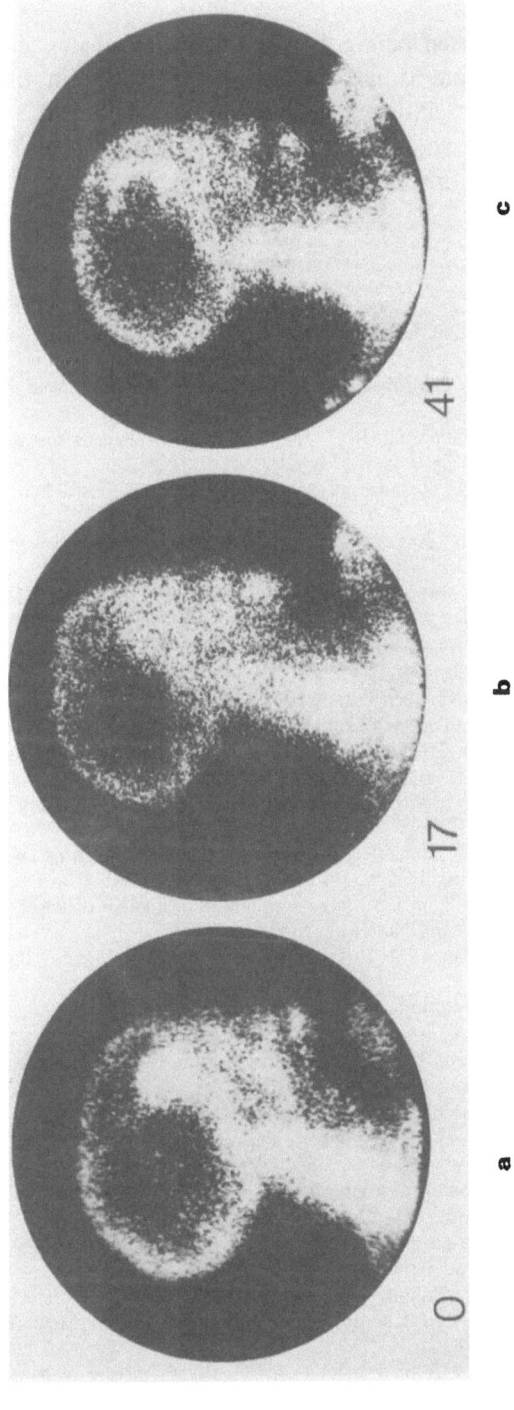

Figure 15a. The round area of increased uptake correlates with osteoporosis circumscripta on the radiograph of the skull.
b. After 17 months of treatment normalization is almost achieved.
c. After 41 months progression of Paget's disease beyond the original borders is apparent. At this time the recurrence was obvious also clinically.

parameters, one being dependent on osteoblastic activity, the other on multiple factors.

Although heavily affected bones show a somewhat greater tendency toward deterioration, there is no prognostic significance in the pre-treatment distribution or scintigraphic severity. Thus neither the rate of improvement nor the chance of normalization nor the chance of recurrence can be predicted from the original scintigraphic pattern.

REFERENCES

1. Paget J: On a form of chronic inflammation of bones (osteitis deformans). Med Chir Trans 60:37-64, 1877.
2. Schmorl G: Ueber osteitis deformans Paget. Virchows Arch Pathol Anat 283:694-751, 1932.
3. Dickson DD, Camp JD, Ghormley RK: Osteitis deformans: Paget's disease of the bone. Radiology 44: 449-470, 1945.
4. Collins DH: Paget's disease of bone: incidence and subclinical forms. Lancet 2:51, 1956.
5. Nagant de Deuxchaisnes C, Krane SM: Paget's disease of bone: clinical and metabolic observations. Medicine 43: 233-266, 1964.
6. Rosenkrantz JA, Wolf J, Kaicher JJ: Paget's disease (osteitis deformans). AMA Arch Int Med 90:610-633, 1952.
7. Gutman AB, Kasabach H: Paget's disease (osteitis deformans): analysis of 116 cases. Am J Med Sci 191:361-380, 1936.
8. Bijvoet OLM, Van der Sluys Veer J, Janssen AP: Effects of calcitonin on patients with Paget's disease, thyrotoxicosis or hypercalcaemia. The Lancet i:876-881, 1968.
9. Franck WA, Bress NM, Singer FR et al.: Rheumatic manifestations of Paget's disease of bone. Am J Med 56:592-603, 1974.
10. Lake ME: The pathology of fracture in Paget's disease. Aust NZJ Surg 27:307, 1958.
11. Knaggs RL: On osteitis deformans (Paget's disease) and its relation to osteitis fibrosa and osteomalacia. Brit J Surg 13:206, 1925.
12. Shirazi PH, Ryan WG, Fordham EW: Bone scanning in evaluation of Paget's disease of bone. CRC in Clin Rad and Nucl Med 5:523-558, 1974.
13. Porretta CA, Dahlin DC, Janes JM: Sarcoma in Paget's disease of bone. J Bone Joint Surg 39A:1314, 1957.
14. Speiser F: Sarkomatöse Entartung bei der Osteitis Deformans. Arch Surg 23:918, 1931.
15. Brailsford J: Paget's disease of bone – its frequency, diagnosis and complications. Brit J Radiol 11:507-532, 1938.
16. Brailsford J: Paget's disease of bone. Brit J Radiol 27:435-442, 1954.
17. Seaman WB: The roentgen appearance of early Paget's disease. Am J Roentg 66:587-593, 1951.
18. Edeiken J, Hodes PJ: Roentgen diagnosis of diseases of bone. The Williams & Wilkins Company, Baltimore, 1973 (2nd edition), p 523-542.
19. Sosman MC: Radiology as an aid in the diagnosis of skull and intracranial lesions. Radiology 9:396, 1927.
20. Bijvoet OLM, Hosking DJ, Frijlink WB, te Velde J, Vellenga CJLR: Treatment of Paget's disease with combined calcitonin and diphosphonate (EHDP). Metab Bone dis & Rel Res 1:251-261, 1978.
21. Khairi MRA, Wellman HN, Robb JA, Johnson CC: Paget's disease of bone; symptomatic lesions and bone scan. Annals Int Med 79:348-351, 1973.

22. Bauer GCH, Ray RD: Kinetics of Strontium metabolism in man. J Bone & Joint Surg 40A:171-186, 1958.
23. Klein EW, Lund RR: Strontium-85 photoscanning in Paget's disease. Am J Roentg 92:195-201, 1964.
24. Altman RD, Johnston CC, Khairi MRA, Wellman H, Serafini AN, Sankey RR: Influence of disodium etidronate on clinical and laboratory manifestations of Paget's disease of bone. The New Engl J Med 289:1379-1384, 1973.
25. Marshall JH: Measurement and models of skeletal metabolism. In: Mineral metabolism, vol III, Calcium physiology, Comar CL, Bronner F (eds), New York, Academic Press, 1969, p 1-122.
26. Goldman AB, Braunstein P, Wilkinson D, Kammerman S: Radionuclide uptake studies of bone: a quantitative method of evaluating the response of patients with Paget's disease to diphosphonate therapy. Radiology 117:365-369, 1975.
27. Stein I, Shapiro B, Ostrum B, Beller ML: Evaluation of sodium etidronate in the treatment of Paget's disease of bone. Clin Orthopaedics and Rel Res 122:347-358, 1977.
28. Lentle BC, Russell AS, Heslip PG, Peroy JS: The scintigraphic findings in Paget's disease of bone. Clin Radiol 27:129-135, 1976.
29. Waxman AD, Ducker S, McKee D, Siemsen JK, Singer FR: Evaluation of ^{99m}Tc-diphosphonate kinetics and bone scans in patients with Paget's disease before and after calcitonin treatment. Radiology 125:761-764, 1977.
30. Lavender JP, Evans IMA, Arnot R, Bowring S, Doyle FH, Joplin GF, MacIntyre I: A comparison of radiography and radio-isotope scanning in the detection of Paget's disease and in the assessment of response to human calcitonin. Brit J Rad 50:243-250, 1977.
31. Miller SW, Castronovo PP, Pendergrass HP, Potsaid MS: Technetium-99m labeled diphosphonate bone scanning in Paget's disease. Radiology 121:177-183, 1974.
32. Serafini AN: Paget's disease of bone. Sem in Nucl Med 6:47-58, 1976.
33. Vellenga CJLR, Pauwels EKJ, Bijvoet OLM, Hosking DJ: Bone scintigraphy in osteitis deformans before, during and after treatment. J Nucl Med 19:706, 1978.
34. Vellenga CJLR, Pauwels EKJ, Bijvoet OLM, Frijlink WB: Evaluation of therapy in Paget's disease by means of bone scintigraphy. Brit J Rad 52:248, 1979.
35. Vellenga CJLR, Pauwels EKJ, Bijvoet OLM, Hosking DJ, Frijlink WB: Bone scintigraphy in Paget's disease treated with combined calcitonin and diphosphonate (EHDP). In preparation.
36. Hadjipavlou AG, Tsoukas GM, Siller TN, Danais S, Greenwood F: Combination drug therapy in treatment of Paget's disease of bone. J Bone and Joint Surgery 59-A, 1045-1051, 1977.
37. Fletcher JW, Butler RL, Henry RE, Solaric-George E, Donati RM: Bone marrow scanning in Paget's disease. J Nucl Med 14: 928-930, 1973.
38. Jones AG, Francis MD, Davis MA: Bone scanning: radionuclidic reaction mechanisms. Seminars in Nucl Med 6:3-18, 1976.
39. King MA, Kilpper RW, Weber DA: A model for local accumulation of bone-imaging radiopharmaceuticals. J Nucl Med 18:1106-1111, 1977.
40. Genant HK, Bautovich GJ, Singh M, Lathrop KA, Harper PV: Bone-seeking radionuclides: an in vivo study of factors affecting skeletal uptake. Radiology 113:373-382, 1974.
41. Sagar VV, Piccone JM, Charkes ND: Studies of skeletal tracer kinetics, III, Tc-99m-Sn-methylenediphosphonate uptake in the canine tibia as a function of blood flow. J Nucl Med 20:1257-1261, 1979.
42. Rosenthall L, Kaye M: Technetium-99m-pyrophosphate kinetics and imaging in metabolic bone disease. J Nucl Med 16:33-39, 1975.
43. Zimmer AM, Isitman AT, Holmes RA: Enzymatic inhibition of diphosphonate: a proposed mechanism of tissue uptake. J Nucl Med 16:352-356, 1975.

158

44. Rhodes BA, Greyson ND, Hamilton CR, White RI, Giargiana FA, Wagner HN: Absence of anatomic arteriovenous shunts in Paget's disease of bone. New Engl J Med 287:686-689, 1972.
45. Rutishauser E, Veyrat R, Rouiller C: La vascularisation de l'os pagétique: etude anatomo-pathologique. Presse Méd 62:654, 1954.
46. Wallach S, Avramides A, Flores A, Bellavia J, Cohn S: Skeletal turnover and total body elemental composition during extended calcitonin treatment of Paget's disease. Metabolism 24:745-753, 1975.
47. Wootton R: The single-passage extraction of ^{18}F in rabbit bone. Clin Sci Molec Med 47:73-77, 1974.
48. Blau M, Ganatra R, Bender MA: ^{18}F-fluoride for bone imaging. Semin Nucl Med 2:31-37, 1972.
49. Charkes ND, Makler PT jr, Philips C: Studies of skeletal tracer kinetics, 1, Digital-computer solution of a five-compartment model of (^{18}F) fluoride kinetics in humans. J Nucl Med 19:1301-1309, 1978.
50. Charkes ND, Brookes M, Makler PT: Studies of skeletal tracer kinetics, II, Evaluation of a five-compartment model of (^{18}F) fluoride kinetics in rats. J Nucl Med 20:1150-1157, 1979.
51. Vellenga CJLR, Pauwels EKJ, Frijlink WB, Bijvoet OLM: Correlation of radiological and scintigraphic images in untreated Paget's disease. In preparation.
52. Grainger RG, Laws JW: Paget's disease – active or quiescent? Brit J Radiol 30:120-124, 1957.
53. Khairi MRA, Robb JA, Wellman HN, Johnston CC: Radiographs and scans in diagnosing symptomatic lesions of Paget's disease of bone. Geriatrics 29:49-54, 1974.
54. De Rose J, Singer FR, Avramides A, Flores A, Dziadiw R, Baker RK, Wallach S: Response of Paget's disease to porcine and salmon calcitonins. Am J Med 56:858-866, 1974.
55. Woodhouse NJY, Chalmers AH, Wells IP, Dewbury KC, Mohamedally SN: Paget's disease, radiological changes occurring in untreated patients and those on therapy with salmon calcitonin during two years observation. Brit J Rad 50:699-705, 1977.
56. Smith R, Russell RGG, Bishop MC, Woods CG, Bishop M: Paget's disease of bone; experience with a diphosphonate in treatment. Quart J Med 42:235-256, 1973.
57. Russell RGG, Preston C, Smith R, Preston C, Walton RJ, Woods CG: Diphosphonates in Paget's disease. The Lancet i: 894-898, 1974.
58. Canfield R, Rosner W, Skinner J, McWhorter J, Resnick L, Feldman F, Kammerman S, Ryan K, Kunigonis M, Bohne W: Diphosphonate therapy of Paget's disease of bone. J. Clin. Endocr & Metab 44:96-106, 1977.
59. Ryan WG, Schwartz TB, Perlia CP: Effects of mithramycin on Paget's disease of bone. Ann Intern Med 70: 549-557, 1969.
60. Doyle FH, Pennock J, Greenberg PB, Joplin GF, MacIntyre I: Radiological evidence of a dose-related response to longterm treatment of Paget's disease with human calcitonin. Brit J Rad 47:1-8, 1974.
61. Nagant de Deuxchaisnes C, Rombouts-Lindemans C, Huaux JP, Malghem J, Maldague B: Roentgenologic evaluation of the efficacy of calcitonin in Paget's disease of bone. Molecular Endocrinology, Elsevier/North Holland Biomedical Press 213-233, 1977.
62. Van Langevelde, A. Driessen OMJ, Pauwels EKJ, Thesingh CW: Aspects of ^{99m}Technetium binding from an ethane-1-hydroxy-1,1-diphosphonate-^{99m}Tc complex to bone. Eur J Nucl Med 2:47-51, 1977.
63. Merrick MV: Review article – bone scanning. Brit J Rad 48: 327-351, 1975.

PART IV

BONE SCINTIGRAPHY
IN MALIGNANT DISEASE

11. INTRODUCTION TO BONE SCINTIGRAPHY IN MALIGNANT DISEASE

JOHAN VERMEY

Screening for dissemination of the disease
Determination of the extension of the lesion
Screening during follow-up of the patient

For several years it has been generally accepted that oncology is a separate medical speciality. The complicated approach to diagnosis, and the often difficult decisions in the treatment of malignant disease, calls for teams of oncologists of various disciplines, who can deal with different groups of patients with different sorts of malignant disease. For the patient with a malignancy, the disease is not only a physical, but also a psycho-social, disaster, and the doctors attending the patient have to be resolute about the choice of treatment they propose.

It is very important in the approach to these patients, to decide whether the treatment will be curative, or palliative. Although much standardization in oncological treatment has been achieved, the treatment schemes are often complex because of various factors which may be present. Therefore the management of an oncological patient is practically never a routine treatment.

Health benefits and financial costs are other factors in oncology. In the Netherlands, as well as in other western countries, there is already overspending of national budgets for health care (9.2% in the Netherlands). We have to be careful to control the cost of cancer treatment, which is often excessive. In this respect, the primary diagnosis and staging of the disease are of primary importance. A wrong diagnosis may lead to a wrong treatment, and, in a curable disease, may mean an early relapse and inevitable disability for the patient. As a result much suffering and worry arises for the patient and his family, and expensive treatment and care may be required.

Pauwels EKJ, Schütte HE, Taconis WK, eds, Bone scintigraphy, p 161–165.

162

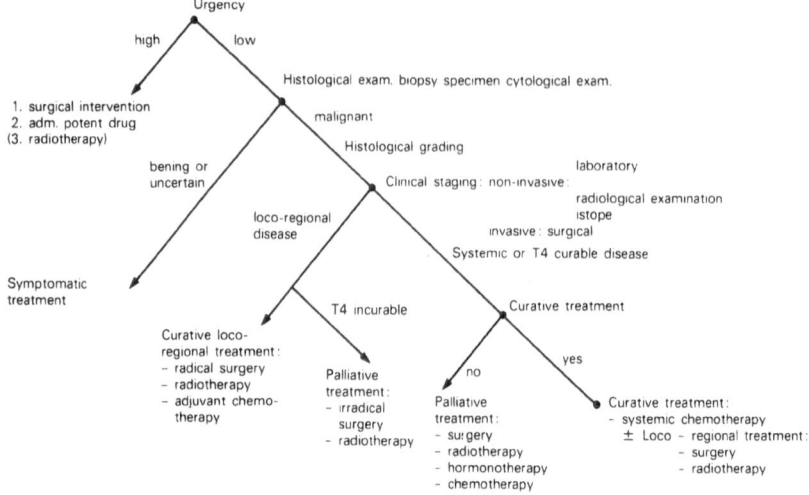

Figure 1. Decision tree: Clinical presentation of patient with likely or suspected malignancy.

1. INDICATIONS FOR BONE SCINTIGRAPHY IN MALIGNANT DISEASE

1.1. *Screening for dissemination of the disease*

This is necessary in the initial examination of new patients or patients with relapse. Decision trees, that lead the way along the various steps of diagnostic procedures, branching off to the different treatment modalities, will give a better understanding (see Figure 1).

Bone scintigraphy has its place in clinical staging and it is obvious that it should be performed in diseases which often cause bone metastases.

Diseases often causing bone metastases:
— prostatic cancer
— breast cancer
— lung cancer (in particular the small anaplastic type)
— thyroid cancer
— primary bone tumours, such as osteosarcoma and Ewing's sarcoma

To a lesser extent:— hypernephroma
— bladder carcinoma
— malignant lymphoma's

In the second group bone scintigraphy should not be performed routinely. In cases of carcinoma, clinical staging will bring clinicians to the decision whether treatment should be curative or palliative. This may mean a great difference to the extent of therapeutic measures. Curative treatment means the utmost effort by the clinician to achieve complete cure, a heavy burden for the patient, and a strong motivation for both. Palliation is the least traumatic treatment required, to relieve symptoms and achieve the best possible quality of life. Therefore the clinical staging should be completed as early as possible in the assessment and treatment of the disease. Bone scintigraphy plays an important role in this respect and moreover it is not traumatic for the patient. The following examples illustrate the influence of bone scintigraphy as well as other clinical examinations on the choice of treatment.

In prostatic and breast cancer, the treatment of the primary tumour, will be influenced if there are proven metastases. Bone scintigraphy may reveal early metastases in these cases. In prostatic cancer with bone metastases, hormonal treatment is given instead of curative radiotherapeutic or surgical treatment. In breast cancer, with proven hematogeneous metastases, a mutilating mastectomy should be omitted and systemic treatment with or without local radiotherapy given.

In other diseases, such as thyroid cancer, bone tumours, hypernephroma and bladder carcinoma, treatment of the primary tumour will be unchanged, but additive chemo-, hormono-, and radiotherapy are indicated, to achieve longer remissions and possibly even cure in the future.

1.2. Determination of the extension of the lesion

Use of bone scintigraphy, may be helpful in primary tumours, when surgical resection is indicated. In secondary disease, bone scintigraphy may be useful to show the extent and number of lesions, especially in the vertebral column, which is of great importance for radiotherapy planning.

1.3. Screening during the follow-up of the patient

In the follow-up of patients with breast cancer, there are various forms of hormonal and chemotherapeutic treatment and the detection of an early metastasis or progression of metastases, is of benefit to the patient.

One should remember that in the first 4 years after initial treatment of the primary tumour, bone metastases will be present in 25% in prostatic cancer, in 34% in stages 1 and 2 breast cancer, in 46% in lung cancer. In Ewing's sarcoma, 55% of the patients will have secondaries within the first two years.

The clinician expects the nuclear specialist to provide objective information and interpretation of the scintigraphic findings, in relation to the patient's history. This interpretation benefits from a good working relationship between clinician, nuclear specialist and radiologist. A particular problem in clinical decision-making arises in cases where bone scintigraphy is the first or only examination suggesting metastatic disease, especially when a solitary spot is observed. Histologic proof by biopsy is not always possible in these cases and close cooperation between clinician and specialists in medical imaging is required to decide whether the hotspot is due to a metastasis or a benign lesion. Up to now, there is no tumour specific radiopharmaceutical selectively accumulating in primary and secondary tumours, which would solve this clinical problem.

In this respect, it would be noted that interpretation of scintigraphic changes during or after therapy in patients with known metastatic disease, is difficult and limited. Future tumour seekers with more specificity for malignant disease, could give more information on the effect of treatment, whether chemotherapy or radiotherapy. It is therefore important to develop tumour seekers, that are detectable in a clinical setting.

In conclusion, it is obvious that bone scintigraphy plays an important role in the detection of secondaries of patients with breast cancer, prostatic cancer and lung cancer, as well as in a number of other malignant tumours, that cause bone metastases to a lesser extent. Bone scans may be useful in measuring the extent of primary bone tumours. It has been emphasized that closer cooperation between nuclear medicine specialists and oncological specialists is necessary to obtain optimal interpretation of scintigraphic images. Further developments in more specific isotopes and tumour markers, will lead to development of further diagnostic facilities and enable assessment of the effects of treatment.

SELECTED READINGS

1. Adams FG: Rectilinear bone scanning: differentiation between metastases and degenerative spinal disease. Brit J Radiol 51:281-285, 1978.

2. Blum RH: An oncologic perspective. Proclinica New York 1979 (New England Nuclear).

3. Dronkers DJ: The detection of tumour metastases in the skeleton with Strontium 85. Thesis, Utrecht 1966.

4. Galasko CSB: The early detection of recurrent and metastatic oncological disease. Proc Royal Soc Med 67:850-851, 1974.

5. Kwang GJ et al: Bone scintigrams: their clinical usefulness in patients with breast carcinoma. Oncology 36:94-98, 1979.

6. McNeil BJ: Rationale for the use of bone scans in selected metastatic and primary tumours. Sem in Nucl Med 8:336, 1978.

7. Mink JH, Bein ME: Diagnostic oncology case studies. Amer J. Roentgenol 130:353-355, 1978.

8. O'Connell MJ: Value of preoperative radionuclide bone scan in suspected primary breast carcinoma. Mayo Clinic Proc 53:221-226, 1978.

9. Woodcock TM: Bone imaging in the oncological patient. Pro Clinica, New York, 1979 (New England Nuclear).

12. A RADIOLOGICAL APPROACH TO METASTATIC BONE DISEASE

Henri E. Schütte

Multiple views
Probabilities
    low probability of having metastatic disease
    high probability of having metastatic disease
    of solitary and multiple lesions to be metastatic disease
Patterns
    the evolutionary pattern
    the photon-deficient lesion
    the benign lesion in the patient with known malignancy
    multiple focal lesions
    problems in decision making

It is well accepted that abnormal tracer uptake in ^{99m}Tc-phosphate bone scans is based on blood flow and bone remodeling and is nonspecific. There are no real specific indicators on the scans that identify a single area as a metastasis and another as a site of benign activity (12). This is who one often needs other methods, like roentgenograms, to collect more information, in order to arrive at a proper diagnosis. All findings must also be interpreted in the light of the patient's clinical history and the nuclear specialist's experience in recognizing the association of certain imaging patterns with specific disease.

In radiological practice, it is accepted to optimize the study to the desired clinical information. Apart from anterior and posterior projections, oblique views and spot films are often desirable. The routine use of imaging tables and traditional gamma camera views may lead to understating certain scintigraphic patterns and/or diagnosing these as metastatic disease (16).

In the following a number of examples illustrate some common difficulties.

1. MULTIPLE VIEWS

1.1. A 53-year-old woman had a routine bone scan as part of her assessment of breast cancer. The left lower ribs demonstrated increased tracer concentration (Figure 1). An oblique scan was done, because the uptake pattern was somewhat unusual, and did not match the anatomical appearance of the ribs. This demonstrated a more anatomical distribution. In fact, three ribs showed focal lesions, instead of the diffused blur formerly seen (Figure 2). This pattern is typical for pseudofractures of the ribs (6).

Pauwels EKJ, Schütte HE, Taconis WK, eds, Bone scintigraphy, p 167–185.

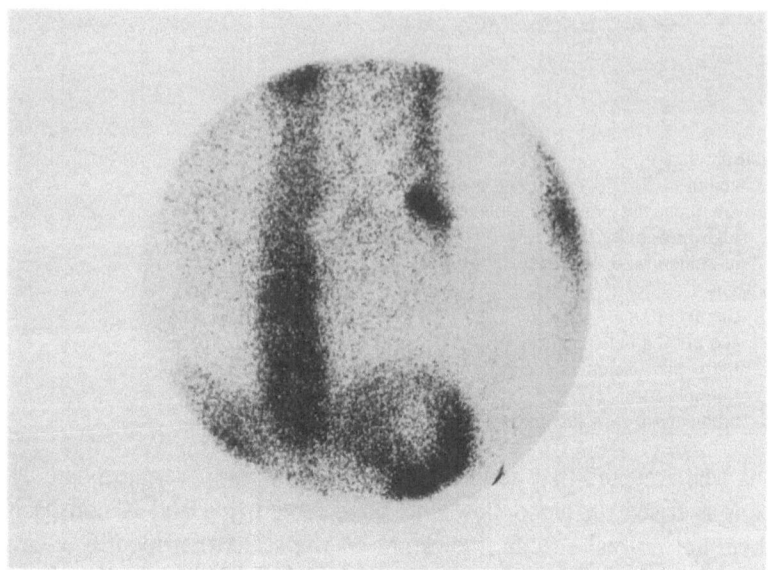

Figure 1. Increased ^{99m}Tc. MDP uptake in the lower ribs, compatible with metastases or artifact. A scan in an oblique position was ordered to rule out the artifact.

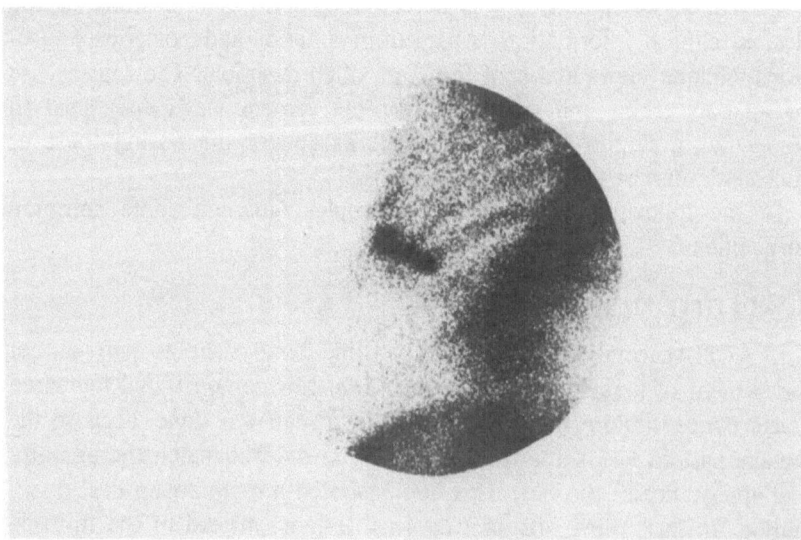

Figure 2. The oblique scan view shows increased tracer uptake in three ribs and this finding now is typical for a linear pattern in ribfractures.

The patient did not complain of pain, but had experienced a chest contusion some months earlier. Had the scintigraphic procedure been done routinely in the anterior and posterior positions, the diagnosis would not have been made so easily. The clinician would have checked the diagnosis with other tests, or more likely, would have diagnosed another stage of malignancy with a worse prognosis.

1.2. Excretion of the tracer into the bladder sometimes leads to super-imposition with the pubic bones. Problems in differentiating between skeletal abnormalities and bladder activity will be greater when the bladder is irregularly filled, or when diverticula exist.

There is a radiological projection described by Chassard and Lapiné and designed for assessment of sigmoid lesions in barium enema studies. For this procedure the patient sits on the table and the sigmoid loops are x-rayed in cranio-caudal direction, resulting in a more stretched sigmoid, without superimposition of the loops.

By having the patient sit on the protected surface of the collimator, the caudal view, analogous to Chassard-Lapiné's projection, provides specific information on bladder activity and increased tracer concentrations in the pelvis, which cannot be separated from each other in any other way (Figure 3).

One must be aware of the effect the weight of the patient may have on the fine lamellae of the collimator. These may be damaged and be the cause of artifacts on the scintigraphic images (Figure 4). We protect the collimator in this position with a firm perspex layer.

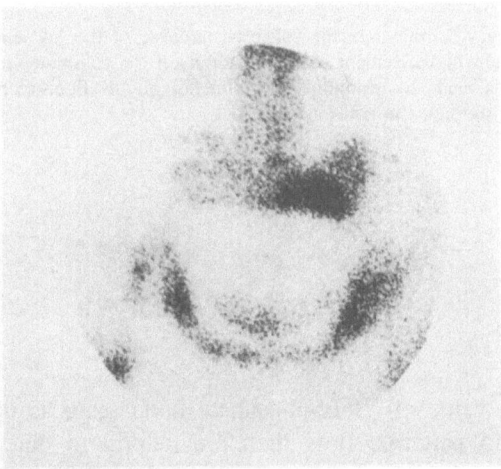

Figure 3. The patient sits on the collimator and this caudal view separates the bladder activity from skeletal structures.

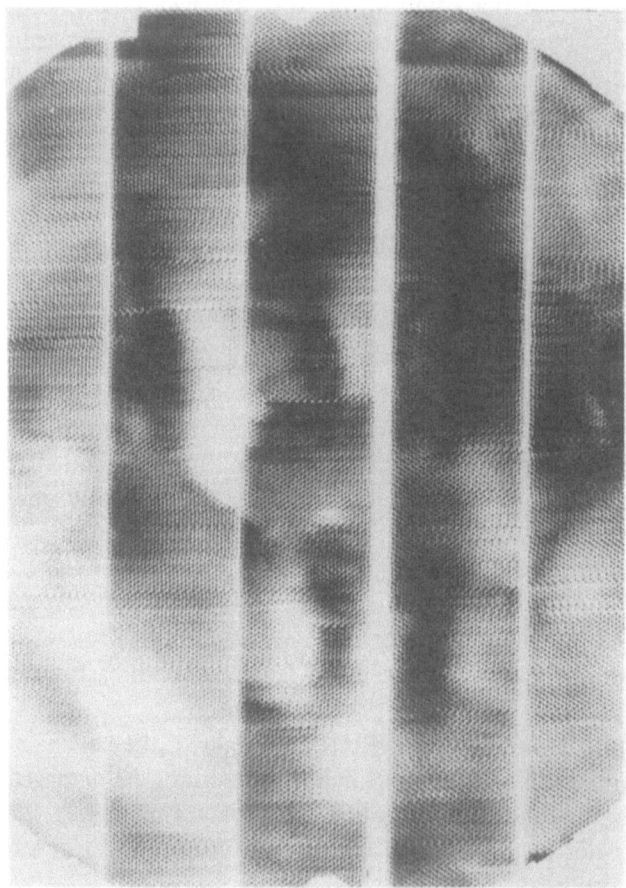

Figure 4. White areas demonstrate the collapsed lamellae of the low energy collimator, caused by the weight of the patient, who had to sit on the collimator for the Chassard view. The film was made by scanning the collimator on the fluoroscopy table, so the x-rayes could pass through the lamellar spaces.

2. PROBABILITIES

The diagnostic value of ^{99m}Tc-phosphate bone scans is dependent on probabilities and patterns. It is therefore helpful to determine if the patient has a high or a low probability of having metastatic bone disease.

2.1. Patients with a low probability of having metastatic disease

In patients with a clinical suspicion of having cancer but without confirmed diagnosis, bone scanning may have only limited value, because a large number of noncancer patients may be in this group. Many isotope laboratories receive patients with bone pain and elevated phosphatase levels for bone scanning and the referring clinician needs to know whether there is a malignant process or metastatic disease present.

We studied a group of 70 patients with bone pain of unknown origin or elevated phosphatase levels, who were suspected more or less to have metastatic disease (15) (see Table 1).

Forty scans were considered negative and these patients remained without malignant disease during the follow-up $1\frac{1}{2}$ years. Bone pain was only temporary and the phosphatase levels returned to normal. Of the remaining 30 patients with positive bone scans, 29 patients were diagnosed as benign or degenerative disease, and Paget's disease. Only one had metastatic disease of the bone, that proved to be a laryngeal carcinoma.

Discussion with the referring clinician as to whether or not to subject these patients to isotope studies was necessary. In case of bone pain, we believe it is better for these patients initially to have the painful area examined radiographically.

Our patient's who proved to have Paget's disease, all had elevated phosphatase levels and we believe that in these cases, when one has a suspicion of dealing with Paget's disease, a bone scan is indicated to assess the different skeletal locations of this disease, instead of asking for a radiological skeletal survey, which may show the lesions less extensive and less early.

When there is very little clinical suspicion of malignant disease the chance the patient may show bone metastases and bone scanning is very low. In our group of 70, only one patient had metastases.

Table 1. Identification of bone pain of unknown origin or elevated serum alkaline and acid phosphatase levels.

Benign conditions	7	Normal	40
Osteoporotic fractures	12		
Metastases	1		
Paget's disease	10		
	—		—
Positive scans	30	Negative scans	40

Schütte. HE: (15).
Cancer 44: 2039, 1979.

172

2.2. *Patients with a high-probability of having metastatic disease*

Patients with advanced cancers have a high probability of having meta-static bone disease. A clearly abnormal study is very likely to be metastases, and lesions with a multiple focal pattern, which has the greatest specificity for metastases, are often present in this group.

Patients with somewhat lower probability than the group just men-tioned, are those with diagnosed malignant disease, but without clinical evidence of metastatic bone disease. Because lung, prostate and breast cancer are known to metastasize readily to bone, patients with this type of cancer often receive bone scans routinely (5).

In practice, a great number of these patients have positive scans not due to metastases, but to degenerative disease. It may be worthwhile to look for indicators to raise the probability in this group of patients in order to minimize the number of negtive scans (see Table 2). Elevated phosphatase levels and bone pain are not reliable enough in prostatic cancer, and in other cancer types bone pain has also proven to be unreliable as an indicator for metastases (11, 13, 17).

Bone pain is caused by: fractures, vertebral collapse and periosteal irritation. If these skeletal causes are ruled out, the pain may be due to radiculopathy, perineuritis and herpes zoster (2). In our practice, bone pain however, proved to be a very good indicator for metastatic disease of the bone.

The results of ^{99m}Tc-diphosphonate and methylene diphosphonate bone scans of 227 of the patients, known to have a malignancy, with and without bone pain are reviewed in Table 3. Fifty-three of the 89 patients with cancer of the breast and persistent bone pain had positive scans due to metastases. In contrast, 60 of 71 without bone pain had normal scans. Two symptomatic patients had false-negative scans, these proved to be lytic lesions, too far from the collimator to be detected or lacking uptake of isotope tracer as described in lytic lesions without reactive new bone (9).

Table 2. Indicators in prostatic cancer.

	Sensitivity	Specificity
Bone pain	53.5%	88.0%
Acid phosphatase	61.5%	89.1%
Alkal. phosphatase	76.8%	87.3%

After Schaffer et al (13) Radiology 121:431, 1976.

Table 3. Bone scan results in 227 patients with known primary tumor with or without bone pain (15).

Primary tumor	Bone pain	Positive scans		Negative scans	
		Metastase	No-metastase	Metastase	No-metastase
Breast	yes (89)	53	20	2	14
	no (71)	7	4		60
Prostate	yes (1)	1			
	no (8)	5			3
Stomach	yes (3)	1			2
	no (1)	1			
Others (colon, lung rectum, bladder, kidney, lymphoma)	yes (37)	27	4	1	5
	no (17)				17

Positive scans interpreted as "no metastases" were diagnosed as benign, degenerative disease and Paget's disease or osteoporotic vertebral fractures. None of these developed metastases in the initial painful area on follow-up for $1\frac{1}{2}$ years. The symptomatic patients without positive scans were analyzed radiographically and the pain was considered not to be of skeletal origin.

However, patients without bone pain, who appeared to have positive scans due to metastases, could be differentiated: 1) in 7 patients with breast cancer, three had lytic lesions, and there was an explanation for the lack of symptoms (15); 2) The other four demonstrated osteoblastic lesions, and radiological signs of destruction or fractures were not present.

All asymptomatic patients with metastases from cancer of the prostate and stomach also demonstrated *pure osteoblastic lesions.*

Naturally, there were also conversions to metastatic disease to the bone during the follow-up time, but these conversions were not considered relevant to our investigation. Various studies have reported the incidence of conversion to metastatic disease in the primary tumors studied (11, 14).

Patients with metastatic disease under or after treatment were not considered in this investigation, because bone pain is expected to decrease as a result of the treatment, and lytic lesions tend to convert into osteoblastic lesions.

In conclusion two indicators for a high-probability of skeletal metastatic disease are shown:

1. known malignancy: 43% of the patients had metastases to bone.
2. known malignancy combined with bone pain: 60% of the patients had metastases, compared to 84% of those without bone pain, who did not have metastases.

In patients with cancer not known to produce osteoblastic metastases, one may wait for the bone pain, which might indicate the presence of metastases and a positive scan. In those with possible osteoblastic metastases, a baseline scan is indicated, in order not to miss the a-symptomatic osteoblastic lesions.

2.3. *The probabilities of solitary and multiple lesions to be metastatic bone disease*

About 6–8% of all metastases are solitary (8). On the bone scan they present themselves with problems. According to Corcoran et al. 36% of the solitary lesions in cancer and non cancer patients are benign, and degenerative, disease (4).

The location of solitary lesions in the skeleton is variable and the prevalence for certain parts of the body is different (see Table 4). There is a 50% chance that a solitary lesion in the skull is a metastasis, whereas in the central skeleton 80% of the solitary lesions might be malignant. In the ribs this percentage is reversed and most focal lesions are caused by fractures (6, 18). In the extremities there is a 40% chance that a solitary lesion is caused by a fracture or a benign lesion like a bone island, e.g. The patient's history or roentgenograms will have to determine the true nature of the scan lesions. Nearly 80% of all meta-static lesions are in the central skeleton, 28% in the ribs and sternum, 39% in the vertebrae, 12% in the pelvis and only 10% are in the cranium and a similar percentage in the long bones (8).

Table 4. Anatomical location of solitary scan abnormalities.

	Extremities	Skull	Axial skeleton	Ribs
Metastases	60%	50%	80%	12%
No metastases	40%	50%	20%	83%

After Corcoran et al (4), Radiology 121:663, 1976.

Even the prevalence of solitary and multiple bone scan abnormalities in noncancer patients is not constant within the population. For instance, ribfractures and osteoporotic vertebral compression fractures are more often seen in older women than in men, in fact, in the age group where metastatic disease is expected.

Primary tumors of the breast and the prostate metastasize predominantly to the central skeleton by way of the vertebral venous plexus (5). Malignant cell groups, more than in other vessels, have the possibility to attach themselves in clusters to the vessel wall, as a result of the very slow circulation in this venous plexus. In contrast, metastases from lung and thyroid cancer generally enter the arterial circulation and may be encountered equally in the central skeleton and the long bones (5, 19).

In conclusion:

1. Solitary lesions in the central skeleton and in the long bones have a higher probability to have a metastatic etiology.
2. Multiple lesions in the long bones and the central skeleton have a greater specificity for metastases.
3. Solitary and multiple lesions in the ribs only, are most likely caused by ribfractures.

3. PATTERNS

3.1. *The evolutionary pattern*

There is a relationship between the quality of scan images and the quality of the radiographic images. This so called "evolutionary pattern", which according to Charkes (3) accounts for over 90% of the focal lesions, can be described in terms of three phases, in comparison with roentgenograms: 1) In de first phase, the scan is abnormal (positive) but insufficient calcium has been deposited in the new bone to be detectable radiographically. 2) Later the scan becomes very hot and the densities are seen by radiograph. 3) Finally the scan returns to normal (false-negative) and the roentgenoggram becomes dense.

This type of evolutionary pattern is also present in malignant bone formation.

In correlating areas of focal accumulation of radionuclide tracer with radiographical findings, different patterns may arise in terms of presentation of disease (10). Pitfalls may be encountered, however, with both techniques and this must be understood.

3.2. *The photon-deficient lesion*

The so-called "cold-spot" or photon-deficient lesion, is a focal decrease of radionuclide tracer in the skeleton, resulting from bone destruction. According to Charkes (3), this mechanism is present in tumor, infection and infarction. The indolent course of bony metastases from thyroid carcinoma associated with low rates of mineral turnover is probably responsible for the low sensitivity of bone scans in detecting skeletal involvement (1). Skeletal metastases from lung carcinoma and also renal carcinoma are known to be very aggressive; the bone destruction may proceed so rapidly that the body's reparative attempts are overridden, and new bone is not formed. As a result of these two mechanisms, photon-deficient lesions may occur, and according to Kober et al. (7) photon-deficient lesions were observed in 2.3% of all pathological bone scans.

Photon-deficient lesions may produce false negative scans, if the "cold-spot" is not recognized on the scan. On the roentgenogram the involved areas almost always are visualized as osteolytic defects. That is probably the reason that the disappointing results of bone scans in multiple myeloma and eosinophilic granuloma, but also in metastatic lesions from lung carcinoma and to a lesser extent breast carcinoma, were considered as a limitation of radionuclide bone scanning, and the value of roentgenographic bone surveys was stressed (7, 9).

But, having recognized the focal areas of decreased tracer uptake, the nuclear specialist may indicate a roentgenographic skeletal survey in order to assess other photon-deficient areas in the skeleton (Figure 5). In this manner, structural details of suspicious areas can be examined. Roentgenograms, however, may also be negative – the main limitation being the failure to detect early lesions, because destruction to some extent is needed for visualization as a defect.

Photon-deficient lesions are seen mainly in the central skeleton and in the pelvis. On the other hand, routine pelvic roentgenograms are often of low quality as a result of faecal superimposition. Bone destruction caused by metastatic disease or primary tumors are often missed on these films. In the radiological assessment of skeletal lesions in this part of the skeleton, one may have to proceed with tomographs, in order to optimize the examination (Figure 6).

Other reasons for the inadequate visualization of, especially, pelvic lesions, and perhaps also lesions in the calvarium, is that the bone structure and the periosteal layers of these parts have little impulses to new bone formation or less periosteal reaction.

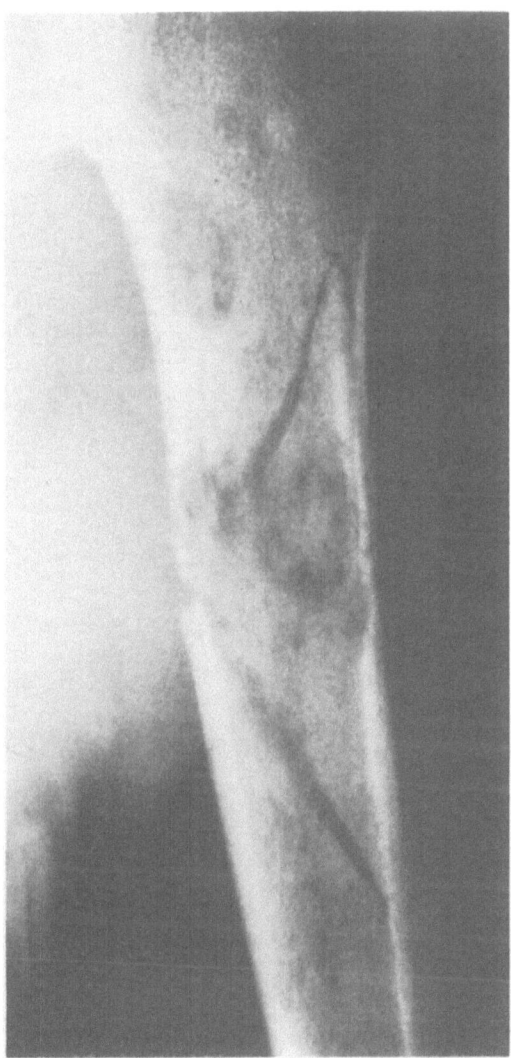

Figure 5a.

Figure 5a, b, c. Roentgenogram of a 40-year-old male patient, who was not known to have malignant disease. There is a very aggressive, destructive lesion, combined with a fracture, consistent with a Ewing type of sarcoma, but because of his age, a metastasis was though to be more likely. A ^{99m}Tc-MDP bone scan was indicated for further assessment and no other focal lesions were seen. Having in mind the permeative destruction of the humerus, the bone scan of the arm was not so metabolically active as expected. In cases like this, the roentgenographic bone survey is very important. The pelvis showed multiple, punched-out lesions, and the final diagnosis appeared to be renal adenocarcinoma with multiple osteolytic metastases to the bone.

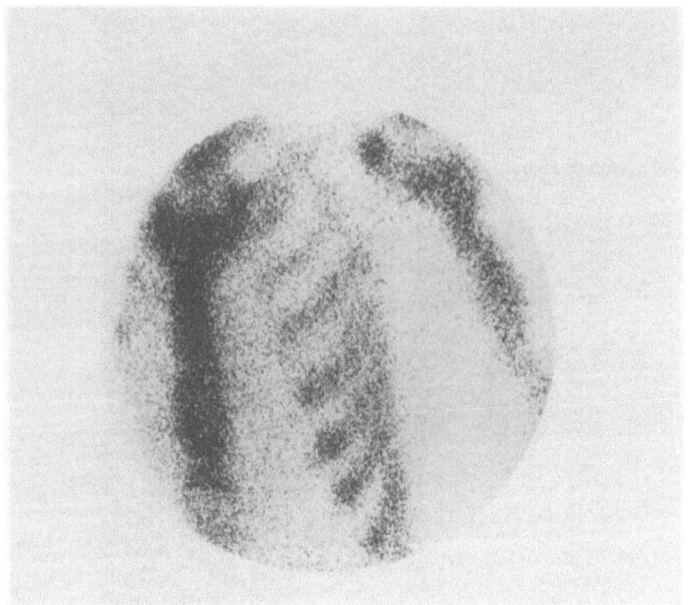

Figure 5b.

3.3. *The benign lesion in the patient with known malignancy*

Some skeletal disorders will have scintigraphic findings, which are easily recognized as a presentation of that particular disorder. The characteristic pattern of Paget's disease, for instance, is a very high tracer uptake, evenly distributed throughout the effected part of the bone, and sometimes with a V-front demarcation. In long bones the tracer uptake may be seen from the epiphyseal part of the bone extending to the diaphysis (see the chapter on Paget's disease in this book).

Other benign disorders may have specific locations, which might be diagnostic, but, in patients known with a malignancy, all these typical patterns will not prevent the nuclear specialist or the clinician from correlating the scintigraphic abnormality with roentgenograms (Figure 7). In certain cases, where even roentgenograms will not bring a solution, because the lesion is not yet visible or difficult to evaluate on the film, the specific scintigraphic pattern of the benign lesion may have a

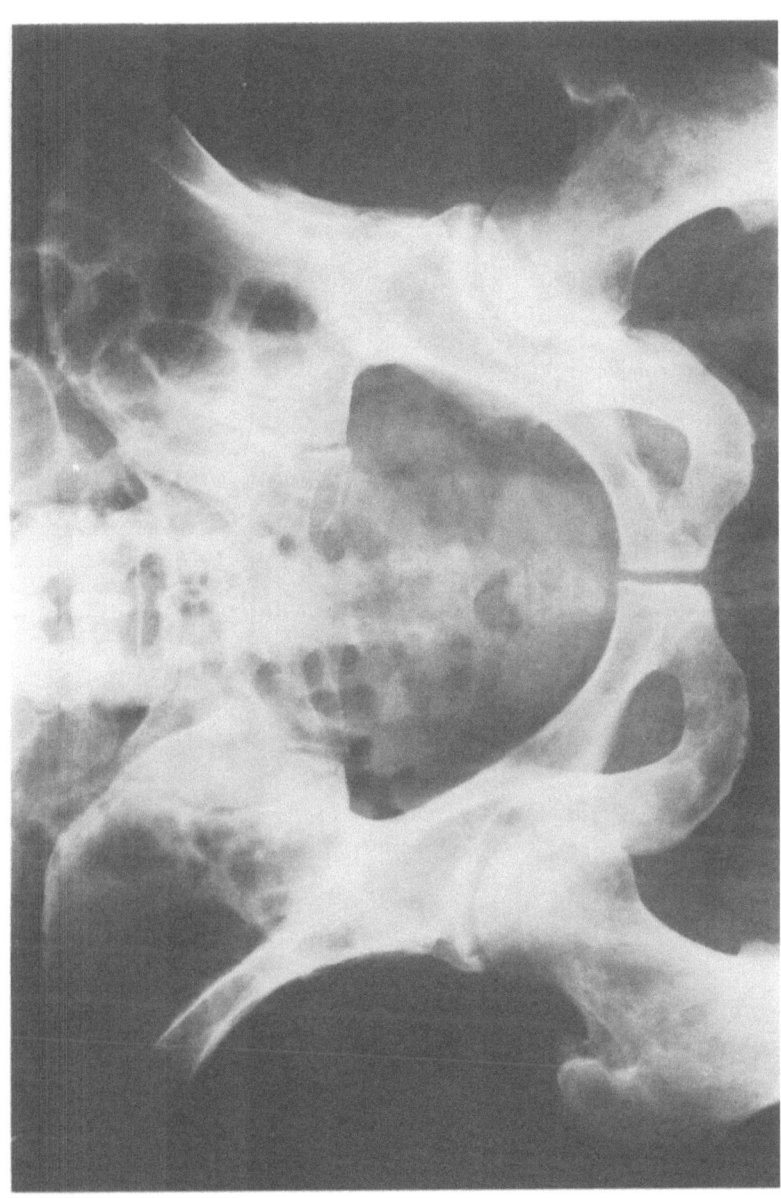

Figure 5c.

180

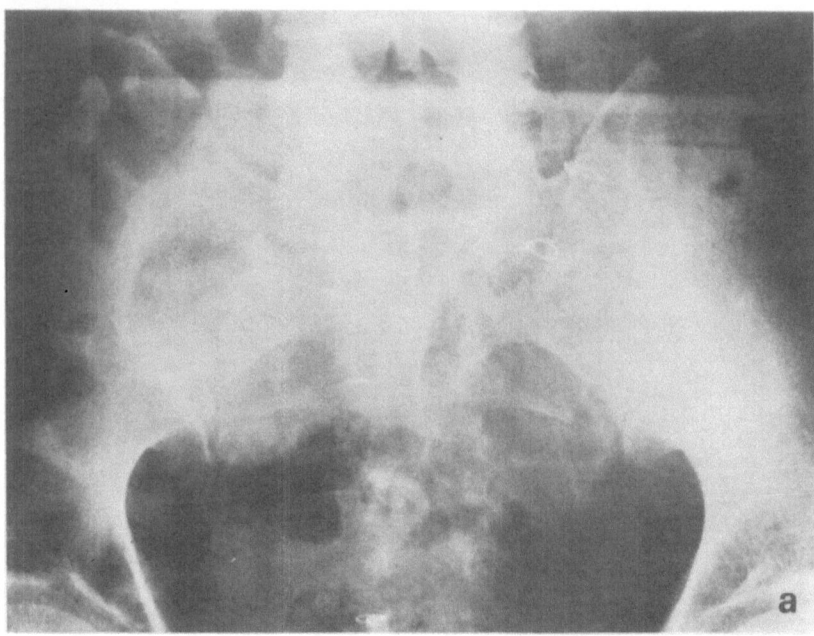

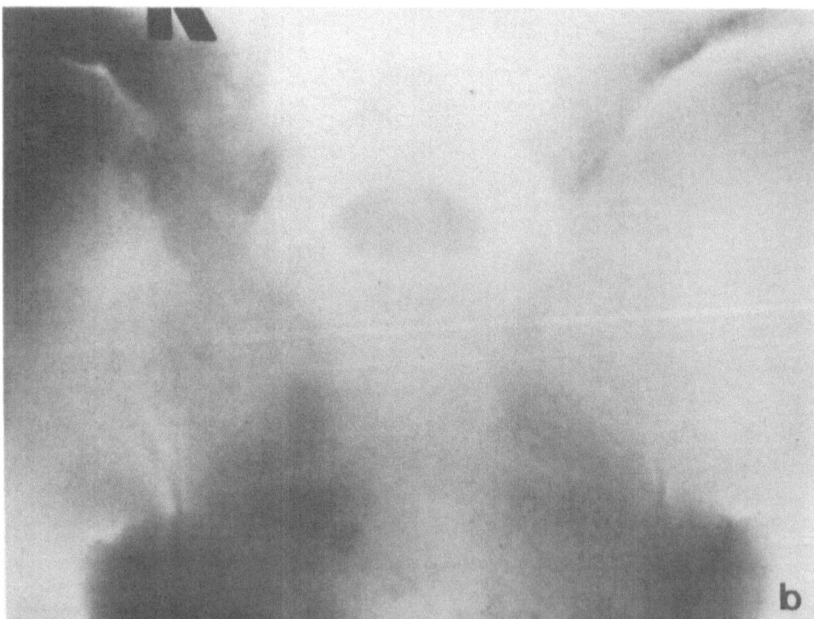

Figure 6a, b. Roentgenogram of a pelvis, made in bed and not under optimal conditions, not showing a lesion in the painful area in the right iliac bone. The ^{99m}Tc-MDP bone scan did show an increased tracer uptake in the sacro-iliac joint.
b. However, on further tomographic work-up the examination was optimized and the lesion clearly seen.

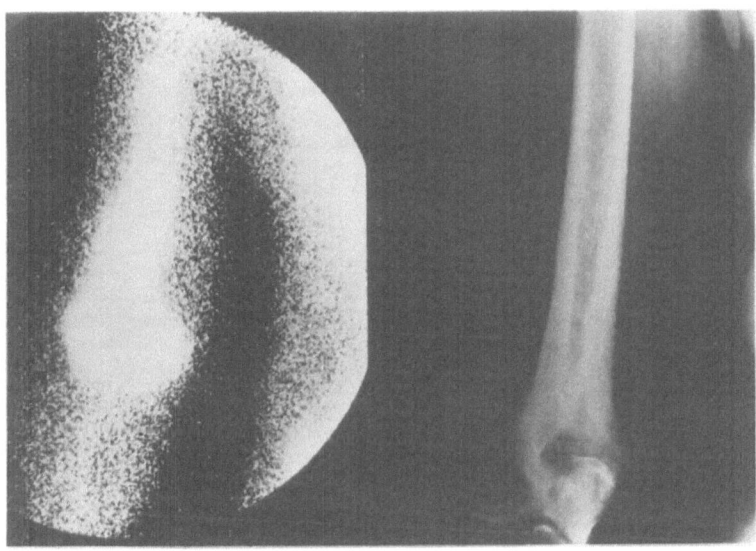

Figure 7. Polaroid film of a ^{99m}Tc-diphosphonate bone scan schowing very high tracer uptake in the humerus, extending from the distal epiphysis to the diaphysis. This pattern is typical for Paget's disease, but nevertheless when the patient is known to have a malignant disease roentgenographic correlation has to be done to be sure.

role in the management of the patient, and biopsies may be postponed.

3.4. *Multiple focal scan abnormalities*

Singh et al. (18) have pointed out that symmetrical focal abnormalities, especially in the femoral necks, ribs and axillary margins of scapulae, may indicate osteomalacia and (pseudo) fractures in osteoporotic bone. These focal lesions may have quite unique patterns, ranging from linear to circular clusters.

When scan abnormalities are seen in the ribs or when they have a symmetrical aspect in the described areas, especially in patients that may have osteoporosis or metabolic bone disease, the pattern must be considered typical for fractures and there is in these cases no need for radiological confirmation.

However, when the focal lesions do also present themselves in the central skeleton, this different pattern is very likely to be metastases (Figure 8). Multiple focal lesions like this pattern, in patients who may

182

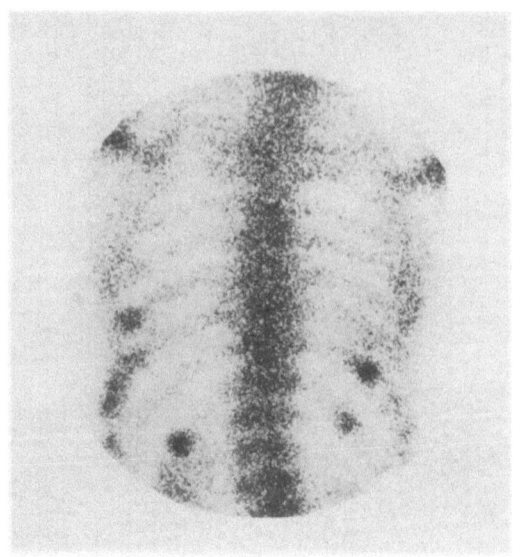

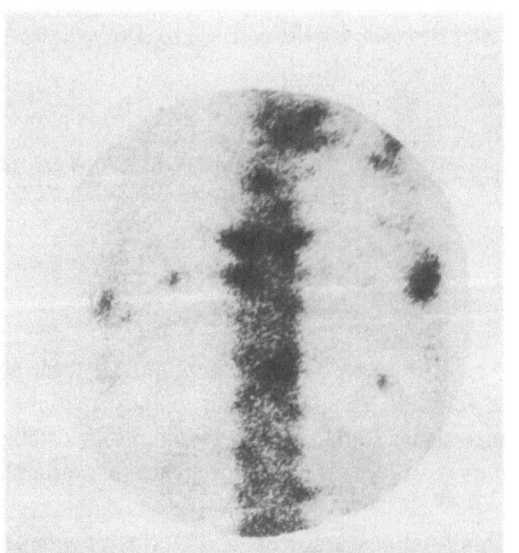

Figure 8a. Multiple lesions only in the ribs most likely are fractures and pseudofractures in osteoporotic and metabolic disease. This is especially the case in older patients and patients who may have suffered a trauma.
b. Multiple lesions in the ribs *and* the central skeleton are highly specific for metastases. The tracer uptake usually confluates in the bones as a sign of progressive growth.

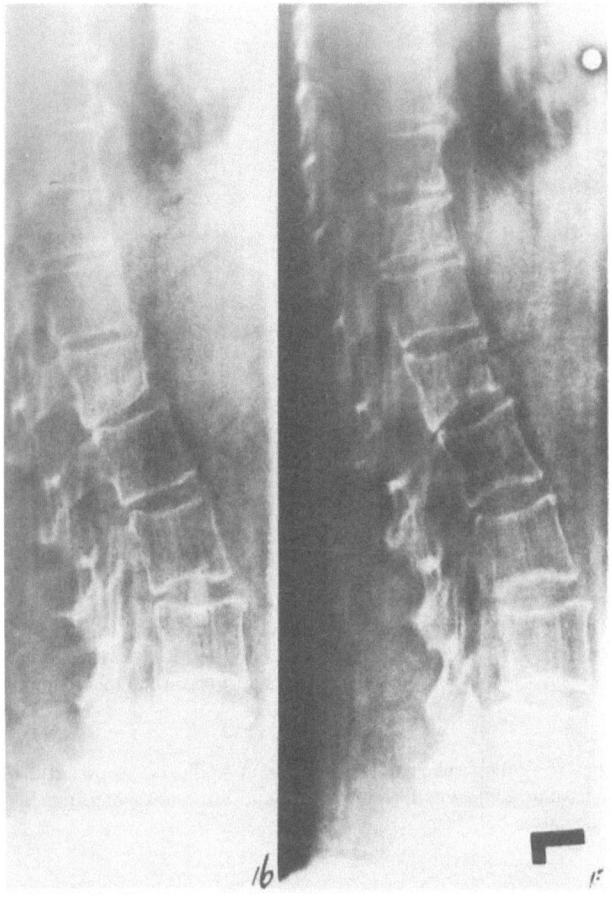

Figure 9a. Osteoporotic vertebral column with compression fracture of a lower thoracic vertebra. Even on roentgenographic tomograms this fracture could easily be caused by the osteoporosis, but still a combination with metastatic bone disease could be present.

have a high probability of having metastatic disease, of course need no radiological confirmation. Only when the distribution of the lesions is very likely to be caused by multiple degenerative disease, may one have to correlate radiographically.

3.5. *Problems in decision making*

Some patterns often present themselves with diagnostical problems. Solitary bone lesions must be considered in this category. In ribs,

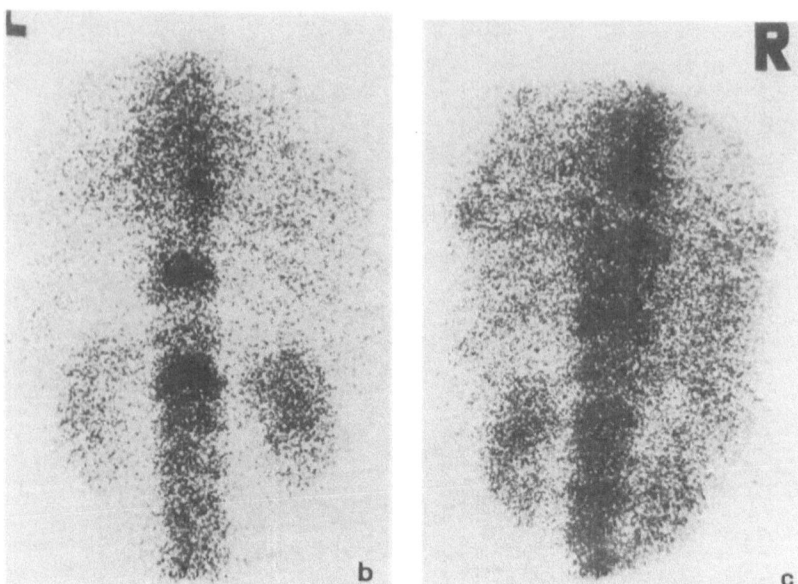

Figure 9b. The ^{99m}Tc-diphosphonate bone scan from November 1974 showed a diffused tracer uptake, with focal lesions. The diagnosis is consistent with the compression fractures in osteoporosis, but to rule out a metastatic origin of the lesions a biopsy is needed.

Figure 9c. The ^{99m}Tc-diphosphonate bone scan from April 1975, shows diffused increased uptake. A metastatic etiology is highly probable and this was demonstrated at autopsy in June to be the case.

sometimes, they will be benign; most of the time radiographs will not be of much help and one has to wait and see what is going to happen, or one has to decide to take biopsies.

It is an unpleasant coincidence that most women with breast cancer are older and may have post-menopausal osteoporosis. The scintigraphic work-up of these patients may produce images consistent with osteoporotic fractures. Even on roentgenograms the proper diagnosis is difficult to make (Figure 9). In the management of these patients, there might be some reluctancy whether to take biopsies, and what has to be done depends on the style and the experience of the clinicians and the clinical picture of the patient. Sometimes these patients will be seen in follow-up with a complete different aspect on the repeat scan. Even if the diffused tracer uptake, and the somewhat faded kidney uptake, will suggest diffuse metastatic disease, the autopsy will have to bring the final "truth"-

REFERENCES

1. Castillo LA, Yeh SDJ, Leeper RD, Benua RS: Bone scans in bone metastases from functioning Thyroid Carcinoma. Clin Nucl Med 5:200, 1980.
2. Charkes ND, Durant D, Barry WE: Bone pain in multiple Myeloma: studies with radioactive 87 m Sr. Arch Intern Med 130:53, 1972.
3. Charkes. ND: Mechanisms of skeletal tracer uptake. J Nucl Med 20:794, 1979.
4. Corcoran RJ, Thrall JH, Kyle RW, Kaminsky RY, Johnson MC: Solitary abnormalities in bone scans of patients with extraosseous malignancies. Radiology 121:663, 1976.
5. Del Regato JA: Pathways of metastatic spread of malignant tumors. Sem in Oncology 4:33, 1977.
6. Fogelman I, McKillop JH, Greig WR, Boyle IT: Pseudofractures of the ribs detected by bone scanning. J Nucl Med 18:1236, 1977.
7. Kober B, Hermann HJ, Wetzel E: "Cold lesions" in bone scintigraphy. Fortschr Röntgenstr 131:545, 1979.
8. Krishnamurthy GT, Tubis M, Hiss J et al: Distribution pattern of metastatic bone disease: a need for total body skeletal image. JAMA 237:2504, 1977.
9. Loeffler RK, Disimone RN, Howland WJ: Limitations of bone scanning in clinical oncology. JAMA 234:1228, 1975.
10. Murray IPC: Bone scanning in child and young adult. Skeletal Radiol 5:1, 1980.
11. McNeil BJ: Rationale for the use of bone scans in selected metastatic and primary tumors. Sem in Nucl Med. 8:336, 1978.
12. Pistenma DA, McDougall IR, Kriss JP: Screening for bone metastases, are only scans necessary? JAMA 231:46, 1975.
13. Schaffer DL, Pendergrass HP: Comparison of enzymes, radiographs and radionuclide methods of detecting bonemetastases from carcinoma of the prostate. Radiology 121:431, 1976.
14. Schaffer DL, Kalisher L: Incidence of bone metastases in women with minimal and occult breast carcinoma. Radiology 124:675, 1977.
15. Schütte HE: The influence of bone pain on the results of bone scans. Cancer 44:2039, 1979.
16. Schütte HE: Some special views in bone scanning. Clin Nucl Med 5:172, 1980.
17. Shafer RB, Reinke, DB: Contribution of the bone scan, serum acid and alkaline phosphatase, and the radiographic bone survey to the management of newly diagnosed carcinoma of the prostate. Clin Nucl Med 2:200, 1977.
18. Singh BN, Kesala BA, Mehta SP, Quinn JL: Osteomalacia on bone scan simulating skeletal metastases. Clin Nucl Med 2:181, 1977.
19. Williams SJ, Green M, Kerr IH: Detection of bone metastases in carcinoma of bronchus. Brit Med J 1:1004, 1977.

13. AN UPDATE ON THE RATIONALE FOR THE USE OF BONE SCANS IN SELECTED METASTATIC AND PRIMARY BONE TUMORS

BARBARA J. McNEIL and JOSEPH F. POLAK

The detection of malignant bone disease has been of interest and concern to physicians for nearly 100 years. In 1889 Paget set the stage for studies involving the search for bone metastases by stating, "The evidence seems to me to be irresistible that in cancer of the breast the bones suffer in a special way which cannot be explained by any theory of embolism alone. Some bones suffer more than others; the disease has its 'seats of election'" (1). Whether Paget was anticipating discovery of the major role of vertebral veins in both breast and prostate cancer is unclear. In any event, his interest and the subsequent discovery of x-rays in 1895 were associated with a surge in the interest in the skeleton and its response to metastatic disease. Nuclear medicine entered this arena in 1942 when Treadwell and co-workers explored the use of radiotracers for studying the metabolism of metastatic bone disease, thus providing the basis of nuclear medicine imaging procedures in the detection of such disease (2). Nearly 20 years later, Fleming et al. performed the first bone scan with ^{85}Sr on a woman with metastatic breast cancer (3).

Their work stimulated a search for better radiopharmaceuticals and imaging devices, and as research progressed through a variety of different bone-seeking radiopharmaceuticals, the radiologic community became preoccupied with determining how often bone scans and radiographic skeletal surveys agreed in their information content and how often they disagreed. The data soon indicated that bone scans were considerably more sensitive, but less specific, than skeletal surveys for the detection of metastatic disease. Today, new areas of research are

Pauwels EKJ, Schütte HE, Taconis WK, eds, Bone scintigraphy, p 187–207.

necessary. It is no longer appropriate merely to develop new agents for bone imaging, to compare scintigraphic and radiographic results, and to describe interesting bone scans. This is, of course, not to say that the more sensitive and specific bone-imaging agents are not needed. They clearly are, as will be seen in the discussion on breast cancer. There, the rapid post-treatment conversion from normal to abnormal scans in many patients suggests that their initial scans may have been false-negative ones.

We must also begin to define the health benefits and financial costs associated with the use of skeletal scintigraphy in patients with malignancies of various sites and stages. Hence, this article will attempt to provide a foundation for the rational use of bone scans in patients with known malignancies. It will be divided into three parts: 1) an enumeration of the anatomic distribution of bone metastases at autopsy and their scintigraphic definition during life, 2) a detailed study of the value of bone scanning in three primary nonosseous and two osseous tumors, and 3) a brief review of the value of bone scanning in a series of miscellaneous tumors for which data are just being collected.

1. DISTRIBUTION OF METASTASES

The maximum percentage of patients having bone metastases that can be detected either initially or during the follow-up of a malignancy is generally no greater than the percentage found at autopsy. For the most common tumors, the percentage of patients with metastases at autopsy is high (Table 1) and undoubtedly accounts for the enthusiasm with which radiographic skeletal surveys and skeletal scintigraphs have been utilized (4, 5).

Nearly 80% of all metastatic lesions discovered during life are in the central skeleton — 28% in the ribs and sternum, 39% in the vertebrae, 12% in the pelvis (6). Only 10% are in the cranium, and a similar percentage is in the long bones, more proximally than distally. It is believed that this distribution may vary depending on the type of tumor present. Primary neoplasms of the breast and prostate often metastasize predominantly to the central skeleton because these tumors frequently are spread by way of the vertebral venous system (7, 8). In contrast, metastases from lung cancer are more likely to involve both the central and appendicular bones equally because lung tumors usually enter the general arterial circulation via the pulmonary veins. Metastases spreading via the arterial circulation should be more randomly distributed throughout the skeleton than are those that spread via the venous

Table 1. Incidence of bone metastases at autopsy in several malignant diseases: general overview (refs. 1,5).

Site of Primary	% Involvement
A. *Common tumors of adulthood*	
Bladder	12-25
Breast	50-85
Hodgkin's	50-70
Kidney	30-50
Lung	30-50
Melanoma	30-40
Prostate	50-70
Thyroid	40
B. *Common tumors of childhood*	
Ewing's	60
Neuroblastoma	80
Osteosarcoma	25
Wilms'	1-10

circulation. In both cases, however, regional bone and bone marrow blood flow, as well as the distribution of red marrow, are probably also important in determining the sites for metastases (9, 10).

About 6%–8% of the time, malignant bone disease appears as a single focus rather than as multiple foci (11, 12). Solitary bone lesions of all causes are generally in the central skeleton (64%). The remaining lesions occur twice as frequently in the extremities as in the skull. Determining the etiology of solitary bone lesions is usually difficult unless a radiograph of the involved region is diagnostic for a malignant or benign process. Otherwise, with the exception of solitary rib lesions, only about 60% (range 54%–64%)* of solitary lesions are malignant; the remaining are the result of trauma or surgical intervention (25%), infections (10%), and miscellaneous etiologies (15%). Therefore, treatment changes in patients with solitary bone lesions should not be made unless the etiology of such lesions is determined pathologically.

2. USE OF BONE SCANS IN PRIMARY AND SECONDARY BONE TUMORS

The use of underlying decision-making processes associated with bone scans in primary and secondary bone tumors can be considered at two

* These numbers arise from two series: one (11) studied 1129 patients all with extraosseous malignancies and observed 172 solitary lesions (64% of which were metastatic). The other (12) studied 100 patients with solitary lesions; the composition of the original population from which these 100 patients derived was not stated, but because of its date (1974) it is likely that most patients also had known malignancies.

points: at the time a patient first presents for treatment and any time thereafter. At both times, three considerations are relevant to rational decision making: 1) yield of abnormal bone scans, 2) assumed health benefits associated with information gained from the scan, and 3) associated financial costs.

In a discussion of yield, it is immediately apparent that the term "yield" without modifiers is not ideal because it included both true positive (TP) and false positive (FP) studies. "True positive yield"* is, therefore, more appropriate. The TP yields for bone scans obtained in patients with all types and stages of tumors ideally should be related to other laboratory, radiographic, and clinical parameters in order to determine the unique contribution of the bone scan.

Health benefits, which occur as a result of information obtained from any diagnostic examination, generally can be categorized in two ways: 1) additional diagnostic or prognostic information available regardless of its effects on subsequent treatment planning, and 2) alterations in mortality and/or morbidity as a result of changes in stage, and hence, treatment. The rationale for performing diagnostic exams for diseases with inefficacious treatments rests on the value of additional diagnostic or prognostic information *per se*. On the other hand, for diseases with efficacious treatments, the rationale rests also on potential reductions in mortality and morbidity resulting from more selectively instituted, or more appropriately timed, treatments.

The impact diagnostic examinations have on total financial costs of diagnosis and treatment is complex and beyond the scope of this discussion. In general, though, any analysis of financial costs associated with diagnostic tests must include not only the cost of testing but also the long-term differences in costs for patients incorrectly treated because of false negative (FN) and false positive (FP) errors of testing.

3. BREAST CANCER

3.1. *Yield*

For the past 5 years, there has been an enormous controversy about the value of preoperative bone scans in patients with breast cancer, with the literature giving a range of positivity varying from under 4% to 38% for patients with clinical Stage I or II (14–35). Recent data suggest that the

---

* Because the true state of nature is generally not known at either presentation or follow-up, it is not possible to determine the true and false positive *ratios*.

Table 2. Data on the yield of true positive bone scans in clinical stages I-III breast cancer (refs. 17, 21, 22, 25).

	True positive bone scans
Clinical stage I	3/150 (2%)
Clinical stage II	4/172 (2%)
Clinical stage III	34/120 (28%)

lower figure is more likely to be the correct one, at least for women in the United States and in parts of Europe (35); combined data from four studies indicate that the yield of TP bone scans in Stage I or II disease is only 2% and in Stage III disease, 28% (17, 21, 22, 25) (Table 2). The average percentage of FP* studies in two of these series was 2% (21, 22). Thus, because the TP and FP yields are approximately equal for patients with Stage I or II breast cancer, pathologic confirmation of metastatic bony disease is essential in these patients.

Follow-up bone scans in patients with breast cancer have indicated that many patients with normal preoperative studies subsequently develop evidence of bone disease (17, 19, 21, 22, 29, 36). This observation is in keeping with the fact that 40%–50% of patients with breast cancer develop their first recurrence in bone (31).

The exact percentage developing metastases is somewhat ambiguous, however, because of small numbers of patients and variable treatment strategies (i.e., some patients with and some without adjuvant therapy). McKillop, Citrin, Kerber, and McNeil all had scintigraphic follow-up in about 50% of their patients and found new bone metastases in about 20%–30% of them in the first 3-4 years of follow-up (19, 21, 22, 34, 36). In one study the time course of the occurrence of metastases was studied and plotted according to standard actuarial techniques (36). It indicated that during the first year after diagnosis there were virtually no *new* cases of bone metastases apart from those seen at presentation. By 18 months, however, the percentage was 15% and by 30 months, 29% (Figure 1). In patients with abnormal scans and normal radiographs, radiographic conversion generally takes place within 12–18 months and frequently (75% of lesions) by 6 months (20).

As expected, patients with advanced-stage tumors and axillary nodal involvement are more likely to convert from normal to abnormal bone scan than are others. In one study, 7% of patients originally stage I,

---

* In this example and in the remainder of the discussion, an abnormal bone scan explained by a benign process is considered a negative scan.

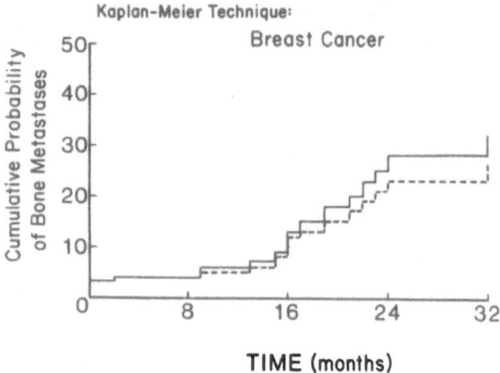

Kaplan-Meier Technique:

Breast Cancer

Cumulative Probability of Bone Metastases

TIME (months)

Figure 1. Probability of bone metastases developing in patients with breast cancer. The solid line represents calculations made using scintigraphic follow-up data only. The broken line represents data calculated assuming that patients had no metastatic bone disease if they were well at the time of clinical follow-up. Both curves are relatively flat for the first year after diagnosis. After 15 months there is a rapid rise in the increase of bone metastases at a rate of approximately 2% per month.
(Reproduced with permission from Radiology 135:174, 1980)

25% of those stage II, and 58% of those stage III converted (22). Moreover, over 2.5 times as many patients developing bony metastases had involved nodes at the time of surgery compared with those who did not (22).

The relationship between the presence or absence of pain and bone metastases is confusing (30, 37–39). In patients on adjuvant chemotherapy, Bonadonna found that 66% of patients with recurrent bone disease had no bone pain; on the other hand, only 30% of patients without adjuvant therapy developed bony lesions without pain (30). In another unpublished survey involving patients *not* on adjuvant therapy at the Peter Bent Brigham Hospital 60% of patients with pain had bone metastases, but 44% of patients without pain also had metastases. Front and his colleagues published analogous data (37), but Schütte found a much greater concordance between bone pain and the presence of metastases (39).

Currently, there are few data on the relationship, either at presentation or during follow-up, of abnormal bone scans to various cancer-associated antigens. However, early results assessing the use of tumor antigens (e.g., CEA) would suggest that they may be a specific (TN ratio = 0.85) but not very sensitive (TP ratio = 0.55) predictor of recurrent disease if CEA levels of more than 5.0 ng/ml are called abnormal (40, 41).

3.2. *Health benefits*

At the time a patient first presents with breast cancer, the discovery of an abnormal scan has significant therapeutic impact in that systemic rather than localized treatment is instituted. If such treatment is incorrect because of a FP bone scan, it is difficult to estimate health sequelae. Similarly, it is difficult to evaluate the sequelae associated with incorrectly administering primarily local treatment because of a FN study. In the latter case, one study may be remotely relevant. Patients who have locally inoperable disease and who are at a higher risk for distant disease have a longer disease-free interval when aggressive systemic therapy is added to local therapy than do those who have local therapy only (33). Thus, it is possible that FN studies may impact adversely on health outcomes.

During the follow-up period, bone scans probably serve their most important role in being a prognostic indicator. Over 30% of Citrin's patients whose bone scans converted from normal to abnormal died in the follow-up period, compared to only 2% of those not converting (19). It appears that scans during the follow-up period could also have impact on health outcomes by documenting early, before symptoms occur, the presence and extent of new disease (42). Resultant treatment could then be more effective. However, there are currently no data to support this hypothesis.

Citrin has summarized potential health benefits from serial bone scans performed on patients receiving adjuvant therapy because of breast cancer (29): 1) identify particularly high-risk patients (43); 2) demonstrate objective response to therapy (42); 3) indicate need for change of adjuvant therapy; 4) provide a rationale for stopping therapy; 5) provide a method for post therapy follow-up, and 6) correlate scan results with other tumor markers.

3.3. *Conclusions*

All patients with clinical Stage III disease should have preoperative bone scans. Because of the high conversion rate after treatment, all patients with Stage I and II disease should have baseline evaluations around the time of their initial treatment. In this group, the etiology of all abnormal scans must be documented pathologically before systemic rather than localized (including adjuvant) therapy is undertaken. Patients should have their first follow-up scan at 12 months and then again yearly in the absence of symptoms or sooner in the presence of symptoms.

Patients undergoing chemotherapeutic treatments as part of clinical trials should have serial bone scans at a more frequent rate in order to create data similar to the information in Figure 1 for patients of varying tumor stages.

4. LUNG CANCER

4.1. Yield

Like breast cancer, the yield of abnormal bone scans in patients with operable (Stage I or II) adenocarcinoma, epidermoid carcinoma, or large cell carcinoma has been controversial (44–48). One small prospective series (52 patients with "resectable bronchogenic carcinoma") had a TP yield of only 2%, and this was matched by an equally large (2%) FP yield (47). Another large prospective series found a TP yield of about 4% in "asymptomatic" patients but this was also matched by an equal number of false positives (52). Other smaller series suggest higher yields – 10% to 35% (53, 54). Autopsy data suggest that such patients with operable bronchogenic carcinoma do have a high prevalence of multiorgan involvement at the time of diagnosis (49, 50). Specifically, distal disease within the thorax (mediastinal node metastases, disease beyond visceral pleura, and infiltration into neighboring structures), as well as liver, brain, bone, and adrenal involvement, occurs in 20%–40% of patients. Thus, yields of occult disease detection in all of these areas are of potential interest.

Follow-up data on the value of bone scans in the post-operative period is limited. In a study by Donato and colleagues, of 7 patients with resectable lung carcinoma and negative radiographs and bone scans at presentation, 3 had positive scans within five months (54). Once a bone scan becomes positive for metastatic disease, the prognosis is grim; in one recent study by Gravenstein et al., for example, it was found that 40/46 patients with positive scans died within 6 months (55).

Gallium scans may be of more use than bone scans in the initial staging of patients with lung cancer because of their ability to detect not only metastases within the skeleton but also those outside. For example, in one study of 61 "asymptomatic" patients with non oat cell tumors, 10/11 patients had distant occult metastatic lesions detected by Ga-67 scanning; four of these patients had osseous lesions also detected by bone scanning (53).

4.2. *Health benefits*

Conventional treatment strategies and their associated health outcomes lend themselves to an evaluation of the impact diagnostic staging tests have on health benefits for patients thought to have operable disease. "Operable" lung cancer is treated with extirpative surgery, which has an average operative risk of 10% (range 5%–20%); patients correctly or incorrectly considered inoperable by virtue of tumor size, location, or the presence of distant metastases, are treated with palliative radiation therapy and, in some instances, experimental chemotherapy. A recent analysis has indicated that the major gain associated with preoperative diagnostic staging tests is a reduction in the number of unnecessary operations and, accordingly, in the number of unnecessary immediate deaths (Table 3)(51). A test with a TP rate of only 50% and a FP rate of 10% would reduce the number of unnecessary operations from 20 per 100 patients to 10 per 100 patients. Depending on the operative mortality rate, the number of unnecessary deaths could be reduced from as much as 4 per 100 patients to less than 1 per 100 patients. Better tests would make correspondingly larger reductions and, in all cases, only small changes would occur in the percentage of patients cured at 5 years. These results take on added importance if we consider the fact that the value of life in the next few years is much greater to some patients with lung cancer than is the value of life 5 years or more hence. Thus, an unnecessary operation and associated perioperative death resulting from failure to recognize distant disease (FN staging test results) may be of even greater importance to a particular patient than the data in Table 3 would suggest.

Table 3. Present health results and health results estimated from use of bone scintigraphy at varying levels of accuracy in 100 patients with "operable" lung cancer (Ref. 51).

	Present results (no scanning)	Estimated results [a] (scanning)		
		TP = 1.0 FP = 0.0	TP = 0.80 FP = 0.10	TP = 0.50 FP = 0.10
# operations performed	100	80	76	82
# unnecessary operations	20	0	4	10
# cured	35.9	35.9	32.3	32.3

[a] These are presented assuming three levels of sensitivity and specificity for bone scanning. Here TP = true positive ratio or the fraction of patients with metastatic disease correctly identified; FP = false positive ratio or the fraction of patients without metastatic disease incorrectly diagnosed as having such disease.

196

4.3. *Conclusions*

Prospective data on the value of bone scans and other staging modalities should be collected in a large number of patients with operable bronchogenic carcinoma. Preoperative bone, or Gallium-67 scans, may be warranted, even if their yield is low, because of the high operative mortality rate in this disease.

5. PROSTATE CANCER

5.1. *Yield*

Metastatic prostatic cancer was one of the first diseases studied with bone scanning and was the source of much of the data comparing the results of bone scanning with the results of radiographic skeletal surveys (55–61). Investigators, however, only recently have become interested in quantitating the value of bone scanning as a preoperative staging modality. The data which are available, however, derive from two studies (66, 67). In one group of 372 patients assessed with serum acid phosphatase, routine bone scan and physical examination, only 53%, 54%, 57% and 26% of Stage IB, II, III, or IVA patients respectively remained in those categories after bone scan, lymphangiogram or pelvic node dissection were performed (66). Both that group (66) and 77 patients in the Cooperative Study of Prostatic Cancer (62), have results similar to those found in patients with breast cancer. In patients with Stage I disease, there is a TP yield of about 5%; for Stage II, the yield increases to 10%, reaching 20% for Stage III. These yields vary with the acid phosphatase level. For example, Paulson et al. observed that in patients with negative radiographic surveys, 17% (33/190) with normal acid phosphatase values had a positive bone scan; when the acid phosphatase was elevated, the yield of positive bone scans increased to 30% (32/97) (66). He also found that patients with negative bone scans and radiological surveys have a higher probability of nodal involvement if their serum acid phosphatase is elevated (62%) rather than normal (25%) (66).

At presentation, the relative sensitivities of other diagnostic modalities, assuming a relative value of 1.00 for scanning, are approximately: skeletal surveys, 0.68; alkaline phosphatase, 0.54–0.77; and acid phosphatase, as determined by standard enzyme assays, 0.5–0.6 (59–61). These results may change when measurement of acid phosphatase is done routinely with the radioimmunoassay rather than with enzymatic

Table 4. Development of metastases at 1 and 5 years by initial acid phosphatase level in prostatic cancer (ref. 63).

Initial phospatase	Percent with metastases	
	at 1 year	at 5 years
≤1.0	3.1	12.8
1.1-2.0	10.5	29.9
2.1-10	20.5	42.0
10+	40.3	66.5

Table 5. Bone pain in reference to scan abnormalities in prostatic cancer (ref. 59).

	Scan +	Scan −	
Pain present	52	9	61
Pain absent	45	65	110
	—	—	—
	97	74	171

TP ratio = 52/97 = 0.54; FP ratio = 9/74 = 0.12.

procedures (64). This latter technique is considerably more sensitive in detecting patients with Stage IV disease than is the standard assay (0.92 versus 0.68, respectively); at the same time, however, its FP component is greater.

Data suggest that the acid phosphatase level appears to correlate with the occurrence of present *or* future bone metastases. In the VA Cooperative Study on Prostatic Cancer, patients with negative skeletal surveys and abnormal acid phosphatase levels (≥ 1 King: Armstrong unit) had a higher chance of developing bone metastases at 1 and 5 years than did those with normal acid phosphatase (Table 4)* (63).

There are no published data on the rate of conversion from a normal to an abnormal bone scan during the follow-up period. Whenever the conversion occurs, however, the first detection of bone metastases is not aided by knowledge of the presence or absence of pain (Table 5): only 54% of patients with bone metastases have pain at this time, and 12% of those without bone metastases also have pain (59). Ultimately, of course, a much larger percentage of patients develop symptomatic metastases.

* In the VA study, patients were initially staged with radiographic skeletal surveys rather than bone scans. Thus, we do not know how many of the patients with metastases present at 1 year radiographically actually would have had scintigraphic evidence for bone lesions at 1 year.

5.2. *Health benefits*

Detection of bone metastases at presentation may make considerable change in the treatment of patients with prostatic carcinoma. Generally, patients with Stage I disease are treated with no therapy, radiation therapy, or prostatectomy; patients with Stage II are treated with radical radiation therapy or occasionally (in younger patients with minimal disease of the well differentiated type) with prostatectomy; patients with Stage III disease are treated with radical radiation therapy; patients with Stage IV disease are generally treated only on onset of symptomatology with estrogens and/or orchiectomy. Thus, abnormal bone scans at presentation may eliminate radical treatment and thus eliminate the potential morbid side effects from these procedures (e.g., incontinence, impotence, GI complications). However, if such scans are FP ones, the consequences are severe, and by eliminating local control, they may eliminate the chance of a cure.

During the follow-up period, early detection of bone metastases in patients with prostatic cancer has no impact on the therapeutic strategy, because data from the VA Cooperative Study suggest that systemic hormonal therapy for Stage IV disease should be reserved until symptoms develop (65). At this point, bone scanning may provide an objective measure of disease remission.

5.3. *Conclusions*

Preoperative data on patients with Stage I, II, and III prostate cancer should be collected. In particular, bone scan results should be correlated with acid phosphatase levels assessed by radioimmunoassay.

6. PRIMARY BONE TUMORS: OSTEOSARCOMA

6.1. *Yield*

During the past 10 years, review of our bone scans in children presenting with osteosarcoma has indicated that approximately 2% of them have distant bone metastases at presentation (68, 69). This figure includes patients with multifocal osteosarcoma.

The widespread use of adjuvant therapy since 1971 has markedly changed the incidence of bone metastases developing during treatment. Before current forms of adjuvant therapy were introduced, about 75%

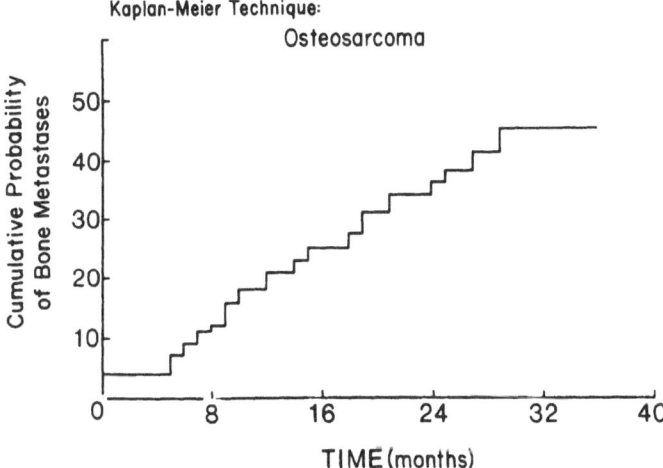

Figure 2. Probability of bone metastases developing in patients with osteosarcoma. There is an almost linear increase in the occurrence of bone metastases between 5 and 29 months after diagnosis; this corresponds to an approximate rate of 1% per month. (Reproduced with permission from Radiology 135:174, 1980.)

of patients developed lung metastases within the first year of treatment and 50% of these later developed bone metastases (68, 70).

The development of bone metastases prior to lung metastases was said to be very rare. Thus, bone scans were utilized primarily to indicate additional sites of relapse beyond the lungs. Our recent experience with patients treated with various forms of adjuvant therapy at the Sidney Farber Cancer Institute over the past 6 years has indicated that 50% of them have thus far developed lung metastases; about two-thirds of these have also developed bone metastases (70). However, approximately 10% of patients developed bone metastases *in the absence of or prior to* lung metastases (69). We noted that few bone metastases were present during the first year after treatment but that by 18 months, 24% of patients had bone metastases and by 30 months 45% (Figure 2)(36).

6.2. *Health benefits*

At presentation, the role of bone scanning in patients with osteosarcoma revolves around better definition of the primary tumor or the identification of distant bone metastases. In the former case, local excisions performed as part of limb preservation protocols are made more precise, and presumably, improved local control should result. In the latter case, there is an enormous impact because of a marked change in type of treatment instituted: an amputation would probably not be performed if bone metastases were identified elsewhere. However, if such bone scans at presentation are FP ones and indicate distal bone disease when there is, in fact, none, then they would have a disastrous impact, and, in essence, would eliminate the chance for a cure.

There are few data relating to early detection of metastatic bone disease in patients with osteosarcoma. However, past experience indicates the importance of early detection of lung metastases: in the absence of treatment of metastatic lung disease, survival at 2 years is less than 10%, whereas with treatment, it is 65% and drops to 40% at 3 years (71). If these data can be extrapolated to patients with bone disease, then failure to detect metastatic bone disease (FN evaluations) may have an adverse effect on survival. On the other hand, FP studies are likely to lead to increased morbidity due to unnecessary aggressive chemotherapy.

6.3. *Conclusions*

All children presenting with osteosarcoma should have a bone scan at presentation to serve as a guide for local excisions, to indicate distant metastases, or, because of the rapid occurrence of bone metastases, to serve as a baseline study. All children with osteosarcoma who are on adjuvant therapy should have follow-up studies every 12 months for the first few years after diagnosis. Currently there are not enough data available to indicate when these routine follow-up scans should stop. If the children are not receiving adjuvant therapy at the beginning of their treatment (a very unlikely occurrence today), scans should be performed only if lung metastases are evident.

7. PRIMARY BONE TUMORS: EWING'S SARCOMA

7.1. *Yield*

Review of our experience during the past 10 years has shown that children with Ewing's sarcoma present with bone metastases more often than do children with osteosarcoma. Three of 28 (11%) children seen in the past 8 years had multiple bone lesions on presentation, and all 3 of these had no evidence of lung metastases (68, 72).

During the follow-up period at the Sidney Farber Cancer Institute, bone metastases occurred in 45% of patients with Ewing's sarcoma. Of these, 38% were detected in the absence of, or before, the development of lung lesions. The median time of occurrence for all bone lesions was 11 months after presentation, and the average time was 14 months.

7.2. *Health benefits*

The role of bone scanning at presentation in patients with Ewing's sarcoma centers around the identification of distant bone metastases. If bone scans at presentation are FP ones and incorrectly indicate distant bone metastases, their effect, as in the case with osteosarcoma, is disastrous. With inappropriate systemic rather than localized treatment, the chance for a cure is eliminated.

During the follow-up period, preliminary data from the Memorial Sloan-Kettering Cancer Center and Sidney Farber Cancer Institute have indicated that vigorous treatment of metastases with chemotherapy improves survival (73, 74). These data would assume a role for early detection of such disease.

7.3. *Conclusions*

At presentation, all children with Ewing's sarcoma should have a bone scan. During the follow-up period, the time course for the development of metastases would suggest at least one bone scan during the first year and another at 2 years.

8. MISCELLANEOUS TUMORS

Quantitative data on the yield of abnormal bone scans in other malignancies graded according to stage and duration of disease are sparse. For completeness, a few recent studies will be mentioned. In 12 patients with *renal cell carcinoma*, all presumably examined at presentation, 5 (42%) had abnormal bone scans (75). In 13 patients with *previously diagnosed colon cancer* who presented with back pain and who were therefore suspected of having recurrent disease, 8 (62%) had abnormal bone scans; the disease in these patients was generally in the pelvic bones, particularly the sacrum (76).

Schechter and his colleagues recently noticed that 2 of 5 patients presenting with lymphoma (Hodgkins's and non-Hodgkins's) had abnormal bone scans and hence were upgraded to Stage IV (77). The yield of

Table 6. Results of bone scan in patients presenting with cervival cancer (ref. 78): Reproduced with permission from Radiology 133:470, 1979.

Tumor stage		Scan findings	
Stage	No. of cases	Metastases	Renal asymmetry
0	3	0	0
I	38	0	1
II	38	0	3
III	11	2	5
IV	3	1	1
"Recurrent"	7	1	1
Total	100	4	11

positive scans for Stage I and II carcinoma of the *cervix* and similar stages of *melanoma* is estimated to be less than 1% (78, 79, 80). In the case of cervical cancer, bone scans have been shown to also provide information about the patency of the urinary tract (Table 6)(78). For example, 43% of patients with either type Stage III or Stage IV cervical cancer had findings suggestive of unilateral or bilateral renal obstruction whereas only 5% of patients with Stage I or Stage II disease had this same finding.

Two studies have recently been published on the role of bone scans in children with neuroblastoma. In the first one, 9 of 12 children were found to have bone metastases, 7 of these were detected scintigraphically; the remaining 2 patients with FN bone scans had metaphyseal lesions (81). The time of bone scanning relative to disease onset was not given. In the second series, approximately the same percentage of patients (29 of 49) had scintigraphic findings consistent with metastases (82). In this study less than 40% of the patients found to have metastases scintigraphically had abnormal radiological examinations. Isotopic uptake by the primary lesion was seen in 35% of cases (82).

9. CONCLUSION

In this review we have concentrated on two areas: the yield of positive bone scans at varying times during the treatment of patients with malignant disease, and the impact such studies have on the therapeutic decision making process. Such a discussion should be immediately recognized as somewhat limited in scope because it neglects three other applications for skeletal scanning: 1) Precise determination of local and distant tumor burden. This could allow more appropriate selection of future types of therapy, viz., immunotherapy and/or combined surgical, radiation, and chemical approaches. 2) Development of prognostic indicators. Although such prognostic indicators may have little impact on the decision-making process of the physician, they may have an enormous impact on the decision making process of the patient. 3) Determination of the natural history of various malignancies under primary and adjuvant therapeutic regimens. This information will be particularly useful in comparing disease-free intervals for new therapeutic approaches.

In general, we know less about the response of cancer patients to treatment than we might because we have not documented in detail the extent and location of primary and recurrent disease. This has been done in the presumed interest of financial cost savings coupled with the attitude "such knowledge will not change any diagnostic or therapeutic strategy; hence, why bother getting it?" Such an attitude is unacceptable today, implying, in essence, that because the medical profession cannot use such information now, it will not need it later. The financial costs associated with the careful documentation of the extent of disease are a fraction of the costs of treating patients with cancer, particularly when patients receive adjuvant therapy every few weeks. Failure to document such disease in a systematic, logical fashion cannot be construed as an admirable attempt to keep the lid on health-care costs but rather as a penny-wise and pound-foolish approach. Of several hundred references on bone scanning in malignant disease listed in a Medlars search, fewer than 20 provide the kind of information needed for rational decision making. The time has long since come for systematic evaluative studies on bone scanning in a variety of malignant processes.

ACKNOWLEDGMENT

We are indebted to Nancy Bernstein and Ellen Zufall, who provided help with data collection from the hospitals affiliated with the Joint Program in Nuclear Medicine, Harvard Medical School.

This work was supported in part by a grant from the National Library of Medicine (NLM 2-9-9569-405).

A large part of this article has been previously published in Seminars in Nuclear Medicine VIII: 336–345, 1978.

REFERENCES

1. Paget S: The distribution of secondary growths in cancer of breast. Lancet 1:571-573, 1889.
2. deG Treadwell A, Low-Beer BVA, Friedell HL, et al: Metabolic studies on neoplasm of bone with the aid of radioactive strontium. Am J Med Sci 204:521-530, 1942.
3. Fleming WH, McIlraith JD, King ER: Photoscanning of bone lesions utilizing strontium-85. Radiology 77:635-636, 1961.
4. Abrams HL, Spiro R, Goldstein N: Metastases in carcinoma; analysis of 1000 autopsied cases. Cancer 3:74-85, 1950.
5. Gilbert HA, Kagan AR: Metastases: incidence, detection and evaluation. In: Weiss L, ed, Fundamental aspects of metastases, Amsterdam: North-Holland Elsevier Excerpta Medica, 1976.
6. Krishnamurthy GT, Tubis M, Hiss J, et al: Distribution pattern of metastatic bone disease: a need for total body skeletal image. JAMA 237:2504-2506, 1977.
7. Batson OV: The vertebral vein system. Am J Roentgenol Radium Ther Nucl Med 78:195-212, 1957.
8. Coman DR, DeLong RP: The role of the vertebral venous system in the metastasis of cancer to the spinal column. Cancer 4:610-618, 1951.
9. Russell WJ, Yoshinaga H, Antoku S, et al: Active bone marrow distribution in the adult. Br J Radiol 39:735-739, 1966.
10. Ellis RE: The distribution of active bone marrow in the adult. Phys Med Biol 5:255-258, 1961.
11. Corcoran RJ, Thrall JH, Kyle RW, et al: Solitary abnormalities in bone scans of patients with extraosseous malignancies. Radiology 121:663-667, 1976.
12. Shirazi PH, Rayudu GVS, Fordham EW: Review of solitary ^{18}F bone scan lesions. Radiology 112:369-372, 1974.
13. Metz CE, Starr SJ, Lusted LB: Quantitative evaluation of visual detection performance in medicine: ROC analysis and determination of diagnostic benefit. In: Proceedings of the Seventh L.H. Gray Conference on Medical Images: formation, perception and measurement. Bristol, UK: Institute of Physics, 1976, pp 220-241.
14. Sklaroff DM, Charkes ND: Bone metastases from breast cancer at the time of radical mastectomy. Surg Gynecol Obstet 127:763-768, 1968.
15. Hoffman HC, Marty R: Bone scanning: its value in the preoperative evaluation of patients with suspicious breast masses. Am J Surg 124:194-198, 1972.
16. Galasko CSB: The detection of skeletal metastases from mammary cancer by gamma camera scintigraphy. Br J Surg 56:757-764, 1969.
17. Baker RR, Holmes ER III, Alderson PO, et al: An evaluation of bone scans as screening procedures for occult metastases in primary breast cancer. Ann Surg 186:363-367, 1977.
18. Citrin DL, Bessent RG, Greig WR, et al: The application of the ^{99}Tc^m phosphate bone scan to the study of breast cancer. Br J Surg 62:201-204, 1975.
19. Citrin DL, Furnival CM, Bessent RG, et al: Radioactive technetium phosphate bone scanning in preoperative assessment and follow-up study of patients with primary cancer of the breast. Surg Gynecol Obstet 143:360-364, 1976.
20. Galasko CS: Skeletal metastases and mammary cancer. Ann R Coll Surg Engl 50:3-28, 1972.
21. Gerber FH, Goodreau JJ, Kirchner PT: Efficacy of preoperative and postoperative bone scanning in the management of breast carcinoma. N Engl J Med 297:300-303, 1977.
22. McNeil BJ, Pace PD, Gray EB, et al: Preoperative and follow-up bone scans in patients with primary carcinoma of the breast. Surg Gynecol Obstet 147:745-748, 1978.
23. Robert JG, Gravelle IH, Baum M, et al: Evaluation of radiography and isotopic scintigraphy for detecting skeletal metastases in breast cancer. Lancet 1:237-239, 1976.

24. Schaffer DL, Kalisher L: Incidence of bone metastases in women with minimal and occult breast carcinoma. Radiology 124:675-680, 1977.
25. El Domeiri AA, Schroff S: Role of preoperative bone scan in carcinoma of the breast. Surg Gynecol Obstet 142:722-724, 1976.
26. Davies CJ, Griffiths PA, Preston BJ, et al: Staging breast cancer: role of bone scanning. Br Med J 2:603-605, 1977.
27. Robbins GF, Knapper WH, Barrie J, et al: Metastatic bone disease developing in patients with potentially curable breast cancer. Cancer 29:1702-1704, 1972.
28. De Wilde A, Frühling J, Osteaux M, et al: Confrontations des resultats de la scintigraphie osseuse et de la radiographie systematique du squelette dans la recherche des metastases au cours de l'evolution des neoplasies mammaries. J Belge Radiol 59:131-138, 1976.
29. Citrin D, Tormey DC, Carbone PP: Implications of the ^{99m}Tc-diphosphonate bone scan on treatment of primary breast cancer. Cancer Treat Reports 61:1249-1252, 1977.
30. Bonadonna G, Rossi A, Valagussa P, et al: The CMF program for operable breast cancer with positive axillary nodes. Cancer 39:2904-2915, 1977.
31. Bruce J, Carter DC, Fraser J: Patterns of recurrent disease in breast cancer. Lancet 1:433-435, 1970.
32. Franchimont P, Zangerle PF, Hendrick JC, et al: Simultaneous assays of cancer associated antigens in benign and malignant breast disease. Cancer 39:2806-2812, 1977.
33. Osteen RT, Chaffey JT, Moore FD, et al: An aggressive multi-modality approach to locally advanced carcinoma of the breast. Surg Gynecol Obstet 147:75-79, 1978.
34. McKillop JH, Blumgart LH, Wood CB, Fogelman I, Furnival CM, Greig WR, Citrin DL: The prognostic and therapeutic implications of the positive radionuclide bone scan in clinically early breast cancer. Br J Surg 65:649-652, 1978.
35. Lindholm A, Lundell L, McArtenson B, Thulin A: Skeletal scintigraphy in the initial assessment of women with breast cancer. Acta Chir scand 145:65-71, 1979.
36. McNeil BJ, Hanley J: Analysis of serial radionuclide bone images in osteosarcoma and breast carcinoma. Radiology 135:171-176, 1980.
37. Front D, Schneck SO, Frankel A, Robinson E: Bone metastases and bone pain in breast cancer: are they closely associated? JAMA 242:1747-1748, 1979.
38. Winchester DP, Sener SF, Khandekar JD et al: Symptomatology as an indicator of recurrent or metastatic breast cancer. Cancer 43:956-960, 1979.
39. Schütte HE: The influence of bone pain on the results of bone scans. Cancer 44:2039-2043, 1979.
40. Falkson HC, Van Der Watt JJ, Portugal MA, Schoeman HS, Falkson G: Role of plasma carcinoembryonic antigen in evaluating patients with breast cancer treated with adjuvant chemotherapy. Cancer Treat Rep 63:1303-1309, 1979.
41. Lokich JJ, Zamcheck N, Lowenstein MW: Sequential carcinoembryonic antigen levels in the therapy of metastatic breast cancer: a predictor and monitor of response and relapse. Ann Intern Med 89:902-906, 1978.
42. Bitran JD, Bekerman C, Desser RK: The predictive value of serial bone scans in assessing response to chemotherapy in advanced breast cancer (AB). Proc AM Assoc Cancer Res 20:1, 1979.
43. Hammond N, Jones SE, Salmon SE, Patton D, Woolfenden J: Predictive value of bone scans in an adjuvant breast cancer program. Cancer 41:138-142, 1978.
44. Operchal JA, Grove RM, Bowen RD: Efficacy of radionuclide procedures in staging of bronchogenic carcinoma. J Nucl Med 17:530, 1976.
45. Grove RM, Christianson RH, Operchal JA, et al: Personal Communication, 1978.
46. Cooper M: Personal communication, 1978.
47. Ramsdell JW, Peters RM, Taylor AT, et al: Multi-organ scans for staging lung cancer. J Thorac Cardiovasc Surg 73:653-658, 1977.
48. Williams SJ, Green M, Kerr IH: Detection of bone metastases in carcinoma of bronchus. Br Med J 1:1004, 1977.

49. Matthews MJ, Kanhouwa S, Pickren J, et al: Frequency of residual and metastatic tumor in patients undergoing curative surgical resection for lung cancer. Cancer Chemother Rep 4:63-67, 1973.

50. Naruke T, Suemasu K, Ishikawa S: Surgical treatment for lung cancer with metastasis to mediastinal lymph nodes. J Thorac Cardiovasc Surg 71:279-285, 1976.

51. McNeil BJ, Collins JJ, Adelstein SJ: Rationale for seeking occult metastases in patients with bronchial carcinoma. Surg Gynecol Obstet 144:389-393, 1977.

52. Hooper RG, Beechler CR, Johnson MC: Radioisotope scanning in initial staging of bronchogenic carcinoma. Am Rev Respir Dis 118:279-286, 1978.

53. Demeester TR, Golomb HM, Kirchner P, Rezai-Zadeh K, Bitran JD, Streete DL, Hoffman PC, Cooper M: The role of gallium-67 scanning in the clinical staging and preoperative evaluation of patients with carcinoma of the lung. Ann Thorac Surg 28:451-464, 1979.

54. Donato AT, Ammerman EG, Sullesta O: Bone scanning in the evaluation of patients with lung cancer. Ann Thorac Surg 27:300-304, 1979.

55. Gravenstein S, Peltz MA, Pories W: How ominous is an abnormal scan in bronchogenic carcinoma? JAMA 241:2523-2524, 1979.

56. Faber DD, Wahman GE, Bailey TA, et al: An evaluation of the strontium-85 scan for the detection and localization of bone metastases from prostatic carcinoma: a preliminary report of 93 cases. J Urol 97:526-532, 1967.

57. Gursel EO, Rezvan M, Sy FA, et al: Comparative evaluation of bone marrow acid phosphatase and bone scanning in staging of prostatic cancer. J Urol 111:53-57, 1974.

58. Marks DS, Eyler WR: Radionuclide bone imaging in the evaluation of prostatic cancer. Henry Ford Hosp Med J 23:161-168, 1975.

59. Schaffer DL, Pendergrass HP: Comparison of enzyme, clinical, radiographic and radionuclide methods of detecting bone metastases from carcinoma of the prostate. Radiology 121:431-434, 1976.

60. Shafer RB, Reinke DB: Contribution of the bone scan, serum acid and alkaline phosphatase, and radiographic bone screening to the management of newly-diagnosed carcinoma of the prostate. J Nucl Med 18:605, 1976.

61. Shafer RB, Reinke DB: Contribution of the bone scan, serum acid and alkaline phosphatase, and the radiographic bone survey to the management of newly-diagnosed carcinoma of the prostate. Clin Nucl Med 2:200, 1977.

62. Shafer RB: Personal communication, 1977.

63. Veterans Administration Cooperative Urological Research Group, Unpublished data, 1976.

64. Foti AG, Cooper JF, Herschman H, et al: Detection of prostatic cancer by solid-phase radioimmunoassay of serum prostatic acid phosphatase. N Engl J Med 297:1357-1361, 1977.

65. Byar DP. Proceedings: The Veterans Administration Cooperative Urological Research Group's studies of cancer of the prostate. Cancer 32:1126-1130, 1973.

66. Paulson DF and Uro-Oncology Research Group: The impact of current staging procedures in assessing disease extent of prostatic adenocarcinoma. J Urol 121:300-302, 1979.

67. Housepian JA, Byar DP, the VA Cooperative Urological Research Group: Quantitative radiology for staging and prognosis of patients with advanced prostatic carcinoma. Urology 14:145-150, 1979.

68. McNeil BJ, Cassady JR, Geiser CF, et al: Fluorine-18 bone scintigraphy in children with osteoscarcoma or Ewing's sarcoma. Radiology 109:627-631, 1973.

69. Goldstein HA, McNeil BJ, Zufall E, et al: Changing indications for bone scintigraphy in patients with osteosarcoma. Radiology 135:177-180, 1980.

70. Jaffe N, Traggis D, Cassady JR, et al: The role of high-dose methotrexate with citrovorum factor "rescue" in the treatment of osteogenic sarcoma. Int J Radiat Oncol Biol Phys 2:261-266, 1977.

71. Jaffe N, Traggis D, Cassady JR, et al: Multi-disciplinary treatment for macrometastatic osteogenic sarcoma. Br Med J 2:1039-1041, 1976.
72. Goldstein H, McNeil BJ, Zufall E, Treves S: Is there still a place for bone scanning in Ewing's sarcoma? J Nucl Med 21:10-12, 1980.
73. Jaffe N, Traggis D, Sallan S, et al: Improved outlook for Ewing's sarcoma with combination chemotherapy (vincristine, actinomycin D and Cyclophosphamide) and radiation therapy. Cancer 38:1925-1930, 1976.
74. Rosen G, Wollner N, Tan C, et al: Disease-free survival in children with Ewing's sarcoma treated with radiation therapy and adjuvant four-drug sequential chemotherapy. Cancer 33:384-393, 1974.
75. Cole AT, Mandell J, Fried FA, Staab EV: The place of bone scan in the diagnosis of renal cell carcinoma. J Urol 114:364-365, 1975.
76. Antoniades J, Croll MN, Walner RJ; Bone scanning in carcinomas of the colon and rectum. Dis Colon Rectum 19:139-43, 1976.
77. Schecter JP, Jones SE, Woolfenden JM, et al: Bone scanning in lymphoma. Cancer 38:1142-1148, 1976.
78. Katz RD, Alderson PO, Rosenshein NB, et al: Utility of bone scanning in detecting occult skeletal metastases from cervical carcinoma. Radiology 133:469-472, 1979.
79. Thomas JH, Panoussopoulos D, Liesmann GE, et al: Scintiscans in the evaluation of patients with malignant melanomas. Surg Obstet Gynecol 149:574-576, 1979.
80. Roth JA, Eilber FR, Bennett LR, et al: Radionuclide photoscanning. Archiv Surg 110:1211-1212, 1975.
81. Kaufman RA, Thrall JH, Keyes JW, et al: False negative bone scans in neuroblastoma metastatic to the end of long bones. Am J Roentgenol 130:131-135, 1978.
82. Howman-Giles RB, Gilday DL, Ash JM: Radionuclide skeletal survey in neuroblastoma. Radiology 131:497-502, 1979.

INDEX

BOERHAAVE SERIES
FOR POSTGRADUATE
MEDICAL EDUCATION

1. Hemker HC, Loeliger EA, Veltkamp JJ, eds: Human blood coagulation. Biochemistry, clinical investigation, therapy. 1969 ISBN 90-6021-008-5
2. Goslings WRO, ed: Diseases of the gastro-intestinal tract. Some diagnostic, therapeutic and fundamental aspects. 1970. ISBN 90-6021-011-5
3. Haas JH de, Hemker HC, Snellen HA, eds: Ischaemic heart disease. 1970. ISBN 90-6021-012-3
4. Gevers RH, Ruys JH, eds: Physiology and pathology in the perinatal period. 1971. ISBN 90-6021-100-6
5. Elkerbout F, Thomas P, Zwaveling A, eds: Cancer chemotherapy. *Out of print*
6. Stoelinga GBA, Van der Werff ten Bosch JJ, eds: Normal and abnormal development of brain and behaviour. 1971. ISBN 90-6021-099-9
7. Spierdijk J, Feldman SA, eds: Anaesthesia and pharmaceutics. 1972. ISBN 90-6021-125-1
8. Snellen HA, Hemker HC, Hugenholtz PG, van Bemmel JH, eds: Quantitation in cardiology. 1972. ISBN 90-6021-139-1
9. Feldman SA, Leigh JM, Spierdijk J, eds: Measurement in anaesthesia. 1974. ISBN 90-6021-203-7
10. Hemker HC, Veltkamp JJ, eds: Prothrombin and related coagulation factors, 1975. ISBN 90-6021-236-3
11. Went LN, Vermeij-Keers C, van der Linden AGJM, eds: Early diagnosis and prevention of genetic diseases. 1975. ISBN 90-6021-237-1
12. Spierdijk J, Feldman SA, Mattie H, eds: Anaesthesia and pharmacology. With a special section on professional hazards. 1976. ISBN 90-6021-294-0
13. van Mierop LHS, Oppenheimer-Dekker A, Bruins CLDC, eds: Embryology and teratology of the heart and the great arteries. Conducting system; transposition of the great arteries; ductus arteriosus. 1978. ISBN 90-6021-424-2
14. de Wolff FA, Mattie H, Breimer DD, eds: Therapeutic relevance of drug assays. 1979. ISBN 90-6021-443-9
15. Keirse MJNC, Anderson ABM, Bennebroek Gravenhorst J, eds: Human parturition. 1979. ISBN 90-6021-445-5
16. van Oosterom AT, Muggia FM, Cleton FJ, eds: Therapeutic progress in ovarian cancer, testicular cancer and the sarcomas. 1980. ISBN 90-6021-452-8
17. van den Tweel JG, Taylor CR, Bosman FT, eds: Malignant lymphoproliferative diseases. 1980. ISBN 90-6021-451-X
18. Welvaart K, Blumgart LH, Kreuning J, eds: Colorectal Cancer. 1980. ISBN 90-6021-465-X
19. Daems WT, Burger EH, Afzelius BA, eds: Cell biological aspects of disease. The plasma membrane and lysosomes. 1981. ISBN 90-6021-466-8
20. Pauwels EK, Schütte HE, Taconis WK, Ell PJ, eds: Bone scintigraphy. 1981. ISBN 90-6021-476-5